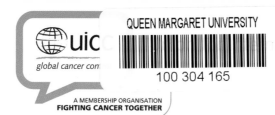

global cancer con

A MEMBERSHIP ORGANISATION
FIGHTING CANCER TOGETHER

:ional Cancer Control

TNM
Atlas

**Illustrated Guide to the TNM Classification
of Malignant Tumours**

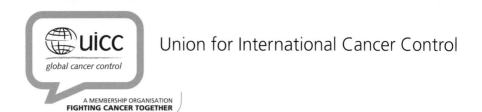

Union for International Cancer Control

TNM
Atlas

**Illustrated Guide to the TNM Classification
of Malignant Tumours**

SEVENTH EDITION

EDITED BY

James D. Brierley
University of Toronto, Canada

Hisao Asamura
Tokyo, Japan

Elisabeth Van Eycken
Brussels, Belgium

Brian Rous
Cambridge, United Kingdom

WILEY Blackwell

This edition first published 2021

© 2021 UICC. Published 2021 by John Wiley & Sons, Ltd This Work is a co-publication between the UICC and John Wiley & Sons, Ltd.

Edition History
UICC (6e, 2014). Published 2014 by John Wiley & Sons Ltd

The right of James D. Brierley, Hisao Asamura, Elisabeth Van Eycken, Brian Rous to be identified as the authors of the editorial material in this work has been asserted in accordance with law.

Registered Offices
John Wiley & Sons, Inc., 111 River Street, Hoboken, NJ 07030, USA
John Wiley & Sons Ltd, The Atrium, Southern Gate, Chichester, West Sussex, PO19 8SQ, UK

Editorial Office
9600 Garsington Road, Oxford, OX4 2DQ, UK

For details of our global editorial offices, customer services, and more information about Wiley products visit us at www.wiley.com.

Wiley also publishes its books in a variety of electronic formats and by print-on-demand. Some content that appears in standard print versions of this book may not be available in other formats.

Library of Congress Cataloging-in-Publication Data

Names: Brierley, James, editor. | Asamura, H., editor. | Eycken, E. Van, editor. | Rous, Brian Arthur, 1967– editor. | Union for International Cancer Control.
Title: TNM atlas : illustrated guide to the TNM classification of malignant tumours / edited by James D. Brierley, Hisao Asamura, Elisabeth Jozefa Van Eycken, Brian Arthur Rous.
Description: Seventh edition. | Hoboken, NJ : Wiley-Blackwell, 2020.
Identifiers: LCCN 2020025431 (print) | LCCN 2020025432 (ebook) | ISBN 9781119263845 (paperback) | ISBN 9781119263913 (adobe pdf) | ISBN 9781119263838 (epub)
Subjects: MESH: Neoplasms–classification | Atlas
Classification: LCC RC258 (print) | LCC RC258 (ebook) | NLM QZ 17 | DDC 616.99/40012–dc23
LC record available at https://lccn.loc.gov/2020025431
LC ebook record available at https://lccn.loc.gov/2020025432

Cover Design: Wiley
Cover Images: (figures) Wiley, (flag) © UICC

Set in 9/12pt and Frutiger LT Std by SPi Global, Pondy, India

Printed in Singapore

M066179_030321

CONTENTS

PREFACE TO THE SEVENTH EDITION

This new seventh edition of the *TNM Atlas* incorporates the changes in the TNM System that are in the eighth edition of the *TNM Classification of Malignant Tumours*.[1] In the eighth edition of the TNM Classification staging at many of the tumour sites is unchanged from the seventh edition. However, some tumour entities and anatomical sites have been newly introduced and some tumours contain modifications; this follows the basic philosophy of maintaining stability of the classification over time. The new additions are: p16 oropharyngeal carcinomas, carcinomas of the thymus, neuroendocrine carcinomas of the pancreas and sarcomas of the spine, pelvis, head and neck, retroperitoneum and thoracic and abdominal viscera. In addition, many tumour sites have important updates.

The Atlas's content follows the approach of depicting the Ts, Ns and Ms in graphic terms. The full-colour artwork is augmented with an increased number of clinical imaging studies illustrating many of the changes between the seventh and eighth editions of the *TNM Classification of Malignant Tumours*.

[1]Brierley, J.D., Gospodarowicz, M.K., Wittekind, C. (eds.) (2017) *TNM Classification of Malignant Tumours*, 8th edn. Chichester: Wiley-Blackwell.

ACKNOWLEDGEMENTS

The editors wish to express their thanks to all who contributed to this seventh edition by comments, questions and their critical interest. In particular we would like to thank Professor Ch. Wittekind, Leipzig, Germany for his enormous contributions as co-editor of the 4th, 5th and 6th editions of the *TNM Atlas,* the 5th, 6th, 7th and 8th editions of the *TNM Classification of Malignant Tumours* and the 2nd, 3rd, 4th and 5th editions of the *TNM Supplement*. He was the driving force behind many of these editions.

The Editors have much pleasure in acknowledging the great help received from the members of the TNM Prognostic Factors Project Committee and the National Staging Committees Global Representatives and International Organizations listed on pages xv–xvi of the *TNM Classification of Malignant Tumours*, 8th edition. In addition, we would like to thank, Dr Brian O'Sullivan and Dr Shao Hui Huang for providing clinical images for the Head and Neck Tumours chapter, Mr Anthony Griffin, Dr Peter Chung and Dr Ali Hosni for providing clinical images for the Tumours of the Bone and Soft tissues chapter and Dr Richard Tsang for clinical Images in the Lymphoma chapter.

This edition builds on the work by contributors to all previous editions. In particular we would like to thank Dr Leslie Sobin and Dr Christian Wittekind, who along with Dr Hisao Asamura edited the 6th edition. Contributors to all previous editions are listed in the 6th edition pp. x–xiv.

CONTRIBUTORS TO THE SEVENTH EDITION

Asamura, H. Tokyo, Japan
Brierley, J. Toronto, Canada
Huang, Shao Hui. Toronto, Canada
O'Sullivan, B. Toronto, Canada

Rous, B. Cambridge, UK
Ruffino, E. Torino. Italy
Van Eycken, E, Brussels, Belgium

Lung
Digestive System, Thyroid, Lymphoma
Head and Neck Tumours
Head and Neck Tumours
Tumours of the Bone and Soft Tissue
Gynaecological Tumours, Skin Tumours
Thymic Tumours
Breast, Urological, Adrenal Cortex Tumours

PRELIMINARY NOTE

The TNM System for describing the anatomical extent of disease is based on assessment of three components:

T – The extent of the primary tumour
N – The absence or presence and extent of regional lymph node metastasis
M – The absence or presence of distant metastasis

The addition of numbers to these three components indicates the extent of the malignant disease, thus:

T0, T1, T2, T3, T4 N0, N1, N2, N3 M0, M1

In effect, the system is a "short-hand notation" for describing the extent of a particular malignant tumour.

Each site is described under the following headings:

1) *Anatomy*
   Drawings of the anatomical sites and subsites are presented with the appropriate ICD-O-3 topography numbers.[1]
2) *Regional Lymph Nodes*
   The regional lymph nodes are listed and shown in drawings.
3) *T/pT Clinical and Pathological Classification of the Primary Tumour*
   The definitions for T and pT categories are presented. In the eighth edition (2017) of the TNM Classification the clinical and pathological classifications (T and pT) generally coincide, therefore the same illustrations are valid for the T and pT classifications for most sites.
4) *N/pN Clinical and Pathological Classification of Regional Lymph Nodes*
   The N and pN categories are presented in a fashion similar to the T and pT categories. Differences between N and pN definitions in the seventh edition arise in the case of carcinomas of the breast and penis and germ cell tumours of the testis.
5) *M/pM Clinical and Pathological Classification of Distant Metastasis*
   M localization is given only in selected cases because of its many possible variables.

Please visit the UICC https://www.uicc.org/resources/tnm/publications-resources or Wiley websites for any errata or updates.
[1] *ICD-O International Classification of Diseases for Oncology*, 3rd edn (2000), WHO, Geneva.

HEAD AND NECK TUMOURS

Introductory Notes

The following sites are included:
- Lip, oral cavity
- Pharynx: oropharynx, nasopharynx, hypopharynx
- Larynx: supraglottis, glottis, subglottis
- Nasal cavity and paranasal sinuses
- Malignant melanoma of upper aerodigestive tract
- Major salivary glands
- Thyroid gland

Carcinomas arising in the minor salivary glands of the upper aerodigestive tract are classified according to the rules for tumours of their anatomical site of origin, e.g., oral cavity.

Regional Lymph Nodes (Figs. 1, 2, 3)

The definitions of the N categories for all head and neck sites except p-16 positive oropharynx, nasopharynx, mucosal malignant melanoma of the upper aerodigestive tract and thyroid are the same.

Midline nodes are considered ipsilateral nodes except in the thyroid.

The status of the regional lymph nodes in head and neck cancer is of considerable prognostic importance. In addition, it is helpful to subdivide the lymph nodes and possible metastasis into specific anatomical subsites and to group these lymph nodes into levels. A consensus guideline from DAHANCA, EORTC, HKNPCSG, NCIC CTG, NCRI, RTOG and TROG has been published and the nodal groups are listed below. However, a number of different classifications exist that use variable level numbers and therefore we recommend the levels be named rather than referred to by number to limit any confusion, although the levels used in the consensus document are given.[1] In the consensus classification, the retropharyngeal nodes are classified as Level VII, but in the classification used by the AJCC, Level VII described the upper mediastinal nodes.

---

[1] Grégoire, V., Ang., K., Budach, W., et al. (2013) Delineation of the neck node levels for head and neck tumors: a 2013 update. DAHANCA, EORTC, HKNPCSG, NCIC CTG, NCRI, RTOG, TROG consensus guidelines. *Radiother Oncol* 2014 110(1):172–181.

TNM Atlas: Illustrated Guide to the TNM Classification of Malignant Tumours, Seventh Edition.
Edited by James D. Brierley, Hisao Asamura, Elisabeth Van Eycken, and Brian Rous.
© 2021 by UICC. Published 2021 by John Wiley & Sons Ltd.

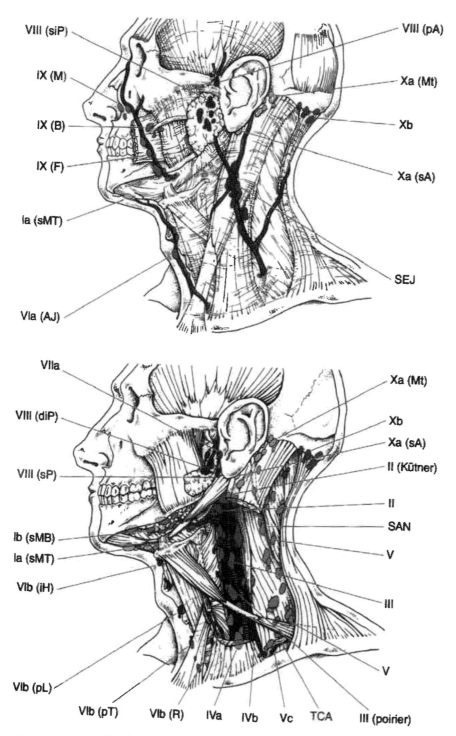

Fig. 1 Source: Modified from Lengele B et al., *Radiothor Oncol*, 2007; 85(1): 146–155.

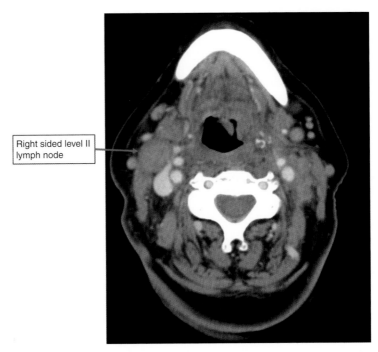

Right sided level II
lymph node

Fig. 2 Axial CT scan showing enlarged right upper jugular (deep cervical) Level II lymph node measuring 2.5 cm in greatest dimension.

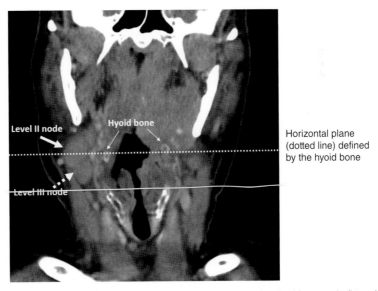

Level II node   Hyoid bone

Horizontal plane
(dotted line) defined
by the hyoid bone

Level III node

Fig. 3 Coronal CT scan showing the same enlarged right upper jugular (deep cervical) Level II lymph node measuring 2.5 cm in greatest dimension, but also an enlarged right medial jugular (deep cervical) Level III lymph node measuring 1.5 cm in greatest dimension. Horizontal plane (dotted line) delineated by the hyoid bone that defines Level II nodes superiorly from Level III nodes inferiorly is marked. This is classified as cN2b: metastasis in multiple ipsilateral lymph nodes, none more than 6 cm in greatest dimension without extranodal extension.

1. Submental nodes
2. Submandibular
3. Cranial jugular (deep cervical) nodes
4. Medial jugular (deep cervical) nodes
5. Caudal jugular (deep cervical) nodes
6. Dorsal cervical (superficial cervical) nodes along the spinal accessory nerve
7. Supraclavicular nodes
8. Prelaryngeal and paratracheal (syn. anterior cervical) nodes
9. Retropharyngeal nodes
10. Parotid nodes
11. Buccal nodes (syn. facial nodes)
12. Retroauricular (syn. mastoid, posterior auricular) and occipital nodes

The lymph node groups are defined as follows
1. **Submental group**
   Lymph nodes within the triangular boundary of the anterior belly of the digastric muscle and the hyoid bone.
2. **Submandibular group**
   Lymph nodes within the boundaries of the anterior and posterior bellies of the digastric muscle and the body of the mandible.
3. **Upper (cranial) jugular group**
   Lymph nodes located around the upper third of the internal jugular vein and adjacent spinal accessory nerve, extending from the hyoid bone (clinical landmark) to the skull base. The posterior boundary is the posterior border of the sternocleidomastoid muscle, and the anterior boundary is the lateral border of the sternohyoid muscle. This group includes the jugulodigastric node, which is the most cranial jugular node.
4. **Middle (medial) jugular group**
   Lymph nodes located around the middle third of the internal jugular vein, extending from the carotid bifurcation superiorly to the omohyoid muscle (surgical landmark) or cricothyroid notch (clinical landmark) inferiorly. The posterior boundary is the posterior border of the sternocleidomastoid muscle, and the anterior boundary is the lateral border of the sternohyoid muscle. This group includes the jugulo-omohyoid lymph node located between the omohyoid muscle and the internal jugular vein.
5. **Lower (caudal) jugular group**
   Lymph nodes located around the lower third of the internal jugular vein, extending from the omohyoid muscle superiorly to the clavicle inferiorly. The posterior boundary is the posterior border of the sternocleidomastoid muscle, and the anterior boundary is the lateral border of the sternohyoid muscle.
6. **Dorsal cervical nodes along the spinal accessory chain**
   This forms the "posterior triangle group". This comprises predominantly the lymph nodes located along the spinal accessory nerve and the transverse cervical artery.
7. **Supraclavicular nodes**
   The posterior boundary is the anterior border of the trapezius muscle, the anterior boundary is the posterior border of the sternocleidomastoid muscle, and the inferior border is the clavicle.
8. **Anterior cervical nodes**
   Lymph nodes surrounding the midline visceral structures of the neck, extending from the level of the hyoid bone superiorly to the suprasternal notch inferiorly. On each side, the lateral boundary is the medial border of the carotid sheath. Located within

this compartment are the perithyroidal lymph nodes, paratracheal lymph nodes, lymph nodes along the recurrent laryngeal nerves and precricoid lymph nodes. Node group 8 (prelaryngeal and paratracheal nodes) may be further subdivided as follows:

8a: cranial paratracheal (suprathyroidal)
8b: thyroidal (perithyroidal)
8c: caudal paratracheal (infrathyroidal, lateral tracheal)
8d: prelaryngeal
8e: pretracheal near the thyroid isthmus (Delphian)

9. **Retropharyngeal nodes**
   These lie in the buccopharyngeal fascia, behind the upper part of the pharynx and in front of the arch of the atlas.

10. **Parotid nodes**
    These may be subdivided into superficial (in front of the tragus on top of the parotid fascia) and deep parotid nodes. The latter are located underneath the parotid fascia and include intraglandular nodes directly in the parotid gland. The preauricular and infra-auricular (infra- or subparotid) nodes are assigned to the parotid nodes.

11. **Buccal (facial) nodes**
    These include the buccinator nodes located deep on the buccinator muscle, the nasolabial nodes located underneath the nasolabial groove, the molar nodes located in the surface of the cheek and the mandibular nodes located outside the lower jaw.

12. **Retroauricular (syn. mastoid, posterior auricular) and occipital nodes**
    The regional lymph nodes for thyroid include the upper (superior) mediastinal lymph nodes, which may be subdivided into tracheo-oesophageal (posterior mediastinal) and upper anterior mediastinal nodes. Cervical and mediastinal lymph nodes are not divided by a fascia; the left brachiocephalic vein is considered as the boundary.

For the tumour entities listed below, a clinical and a pathological N classification have been introduced in the 8th edition of the UICC TNM Classification of Malignant Tumours:

- Lip and oral cavity
- Oropharynx (p-16-negative or oropharyngeal without p-16-IH performed)
- Hypopharynx
- Pharynx
- Nasal cavity and paranasal sinuses
- Unknown primary – cervical nodes
- Major salivary glands
- Skin carcinoma of head and neck

N Classification – Regional Lymph Nodes

N1 Metastasis in a single ipsilateral lymph node, 3 cm or less in greatest dimension without extranodal extension (Fig. 4)

N2a Metastasis in a single ipsilateral lymph node, more than 3 cm but not more than 6 cm in greatest dimension without extranodal extension (Fig. 5)

N2b Metastasis in multiple ipsilateral lymph nodes, none more than 6 cm in greatest dimension without extranodal extension (Fig. 6)

Any head or neck primary except p16-positive oropharynx, nasopharynx, malignant melanoma of upper aerodigestive tract and thyroid gland

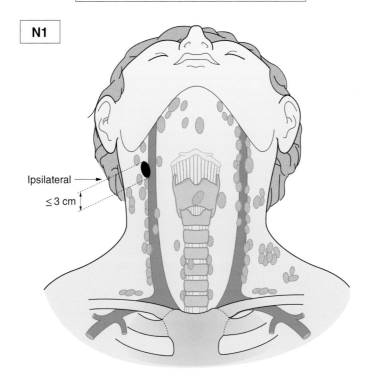

Fig. 4

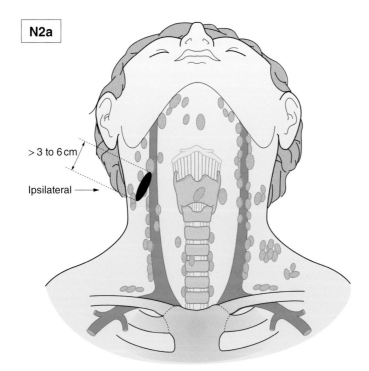

Fig. 5

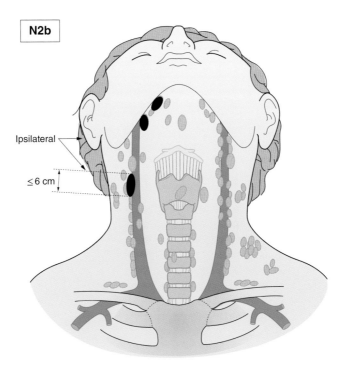

Fig. 6

N2c   Metastasis in bilateral or contralateral lymph nodes, none more than 6 cm in greatest dimension without extranodal extension (Fig. 7)

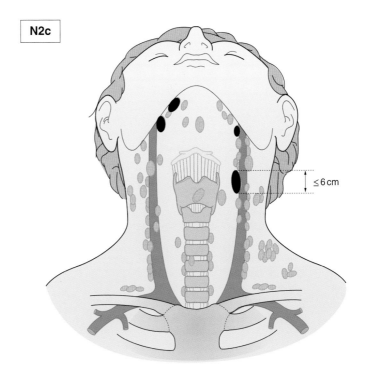

Fig. 7

N3a   Metastasis in a lymph node more than 6 cm in greatest dimension without extranodal extension (Fig. 8)

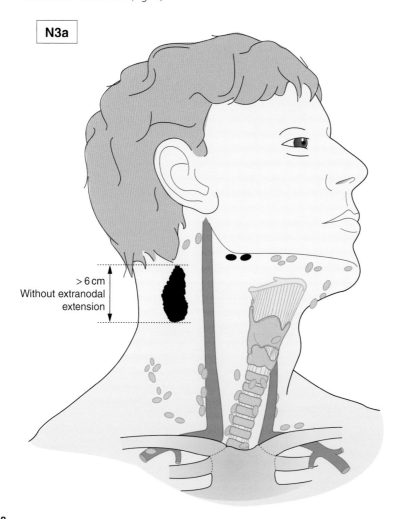

Fig. 8

N3b   Metastasis in a single or multiple lymph node(s) with extranodal extension (Figs. 9, 10)

Note
Midline nodes are considered ipsilateral nodes.

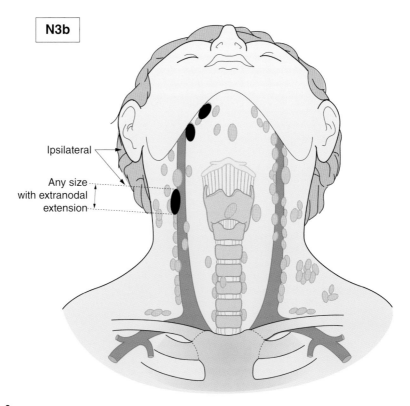

Ipsilateral

Any size
with extranodal
extension

Fig. 9

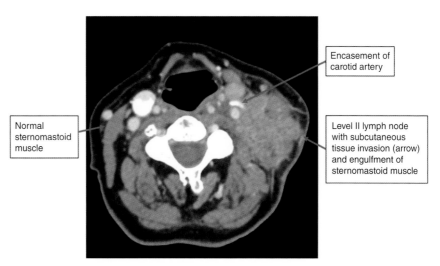

Encasement of
carotid artery

Normal
sternomastoid
muscle

Level II lymph node
with subcutaneous
tissue invasion (arrow)
and engulfment of
sternomastoid muscle

Fig. 10 Axial CT scan showing clinically fixed right upper jugular (deep cervical) Level II lymph node with subcutaneous tissue invasion, engulfment of sternomastoid muscle and encasement of the carotid artery. This is classified as cN3b.

pN Classification – Regional Lymph Nodes

pN0 Histological examination of a selective neck dissection specimen will ordinarily include 6 or more lymph nodes. Histological examination of a radical or modified radical neck dissection specimen will ordinarily include 10 or more lymph nodes. If the lymph nodes are negative, but the number ordinarily examined is not met, classify as pN0. When size is a criterion for pN classification, measurement is made of the metastasis, not of the entire lymph node.

pN1 Metastasis in a single ipsilateral lymph node, 3 cm or less in greatest dimension without extranodal extension (Fig. 11)

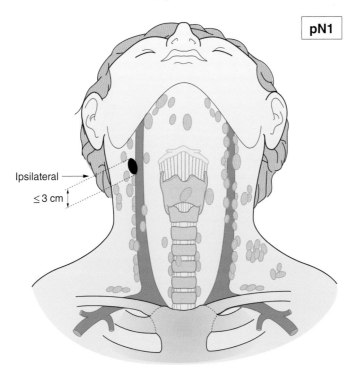

Fig. 11

pN2 Metastasis as described below:

    pN2a Metastasis in a single ipsilateral lymph node, 3cm or less in greatest dimension with extranodal extension (Fig. 12), or more than 3 cm but not more than 6 cm in greatest dimension without extranodal extension (Fig. 13)

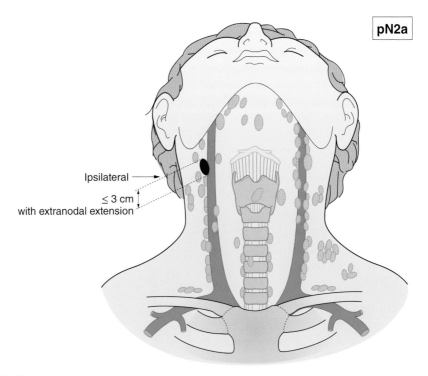

Fig. 12

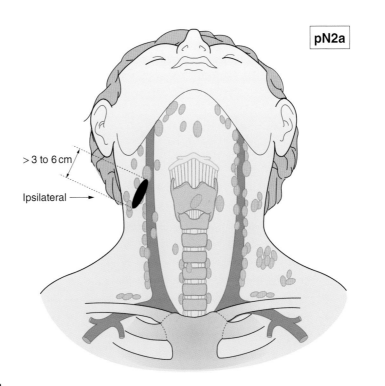

Fig. 13

pN2b   Metastasis in multiple ipsilateral lymph nodes, none more than 6 cm in greatest dimension without extranodal extension (Fig. 14)

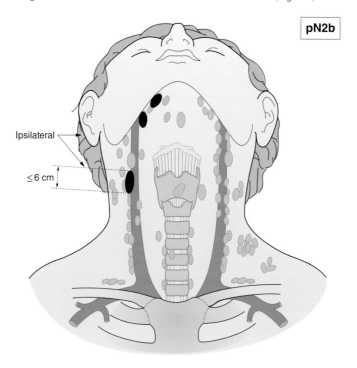

Fig. 14

pN2c   Metastasis in bilateral or contralateral lymph nodes, none more than 6 cm in greatest dimension without extranodal extension (Fig. 15)

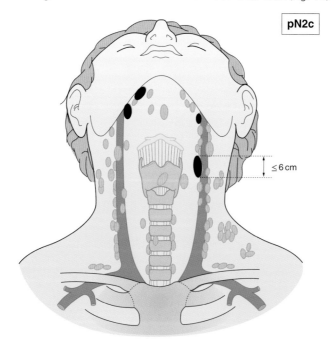

Fig. 15

pN3a Metastasis in a lymph node more than 6 cm in greatest dimension without extranodal extension (Fig. 16)

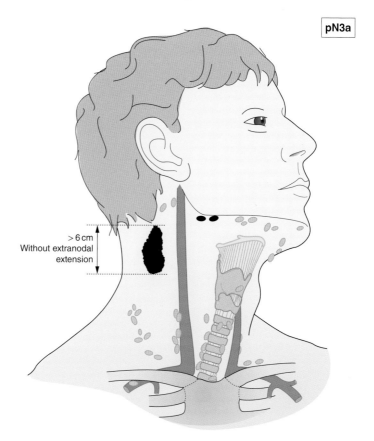

pN3a

>6 cm
Without extranodal
extension

Fig. 16

pN3b   Metastasis in a lymph node more than 3 cm in greatest dimension with extranodal extension, or multiple ipsilateral, contralateral or bilateral with extranodal extension (Figs. 17, 18)

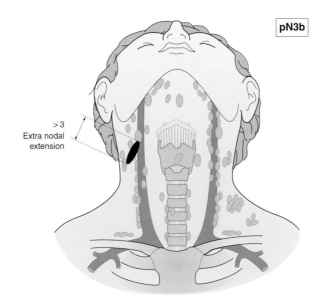

Fig. 17

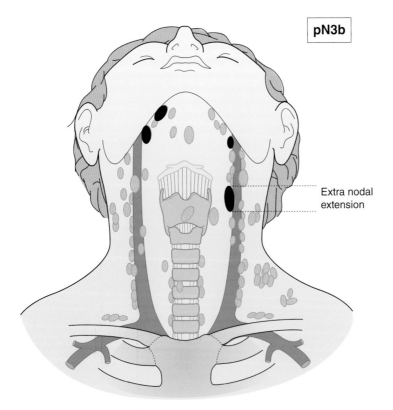

Fig. 18

LIP AND ORAL CAVITY (ICD-O C00, C02–06)

Rules for Classification

The classification applies only to carcinomas of the vermilion surfaces of the lips and of the oral cavity, including those of minor salivary glands. There should be histological confirmation of the disease.

Anatomical Sites and Subsites

Lip* (Fig. 19)

1. External upper lip (vermilion border) (C00.0)
2. External lower lip (vermilion border) (C00.1)
3. Commissures (C00.6)

  * In the 9th edition TNM external upper and lower lip C00.0 and C00.1) and commissure (C00.6) will be classified with carcinoma of the skin.

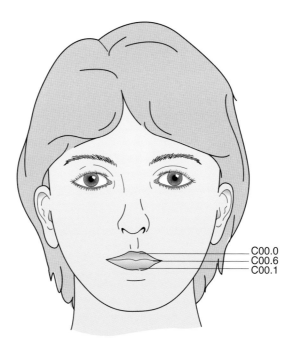

Fig. 19

Oral Cavity (Figs. 20, 21, 22)

1. Buccal mucosa
   (i) Mucosa of upper and lower lips (C00.3, 4)
   (ii) Cheek mucosa (C06.0)
   (iii) Retromolar areas (C06.2)
   (iv) Bucco-alveolar sulci, upper and lower (vestibule of mouth) (C06.1)
2. Upper alveolus and gingiva (upper gum) (C03.0)
3. Lower alveolus and gingiva (lower gum) (C03.1)
4. Hard palate (C05.0)
5. Tongue*
   (i) Dorsal surface and lateral borders anterior to vallate papillae (anterior two-thirds) (C02.0, 1)
   (ii) Inferior (ventral) surface (C02.2)

* Note lingual tonsil, C02.4, is classified in the oropharynx

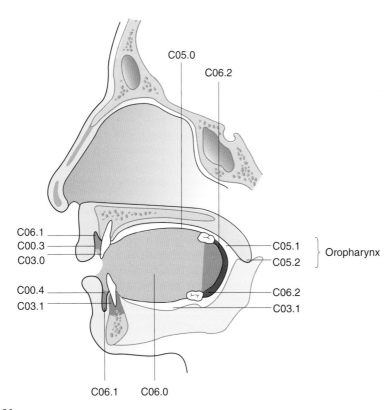

Fig. 20

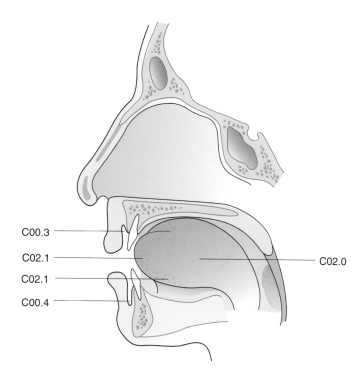

C00.3
C02.1
C02.1
C00.4
C02.0

Fig. 21

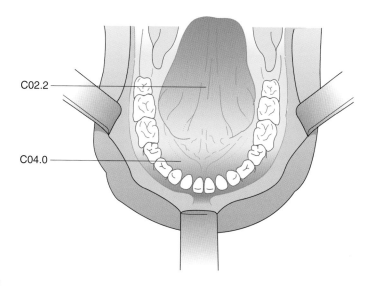

C02.2

C04.0

Fig. 22

TN Clinical Classification

T – Primary Tumour

TX	Primary tumour cannot be assessed
T0	No evidence of primary tumour
Tis	Carcinoma in situ
T1	Tumour 2 cm or less in greatest dimension and 5 mm or less depth of invasion (Figs. 23, 24, 25, 26, 27)

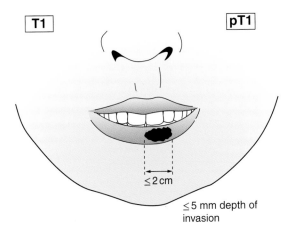

≤2 cm

≤5 mm depth of invasion

Fig. 23

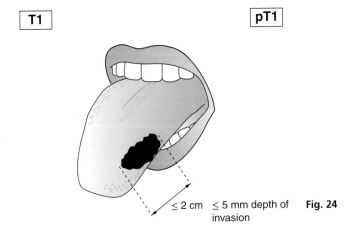

≤ 2 cm   ≤ 5 mm depth of invasion   **Fig. 24**

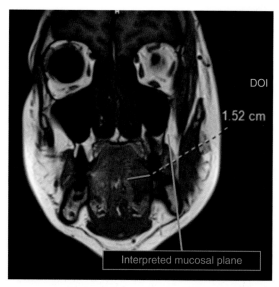

Fig. 25 Example of measuring depth of invasion on a T1 MRI sequence from the mucosal surface to the deepest point of invasion, perpendicular to the interpreted mucosal plane (in blue), a plane just beneath the closest intact surface of normal mucosa for clinical T category.

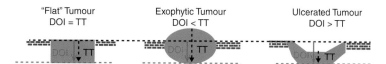

- Black dotted line: IMP ("Interpreted Mucosal Plane"): a plane just beneath the closest intact surface of normal mucosa
- Red solid arrow: DOI ("Depth of Invastion"): measured from IMP to deepest point of invasion
- Black dotted arrow: TT (Tumour thickness): measured from centre of tumour surface to the deepest point of invasion

Fig. 26 Schematic Fig.ure depicting the difference between radiologic depth of invasion (DOI) and tumour thickness (TT) for clinical T category.

T2   Tumour 2 cm or less in greatest dimension and more than 5 mm depth of invasion (Figs 28, 29), or
Tumour more than 2 cm but not more than 4 cm in greatest dimension and depth of invasion not more than 10 mm (Figs. 30, 31)

T3   Tumour more than 2 cm but not more than 4 cm in greatest dimension and depth of invasion more than 10 mm (Figs. 32, 33) or
Tumour more than 4 cm in greatest dimension and not more than 10 mm depth of invasion
(Figs. 34, 35)

T4a   (lip and oral cavity)
Tumour more than 4 cm in greatest dimension and more than 10 mm depth of invasion (Fig. 36), or
(Lip) – Tumour invades through cortical bone, inferior alveolar nerve, floor of mouth or skin (of the chin or the nose) (Figs. 37, 38)

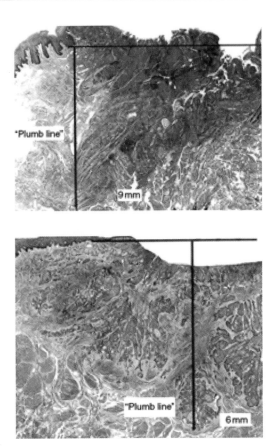

Fig. 27   Measurement of depth of invasion in carcinomas of the oral cavity to assess the pT category. The horizon is established at the level of the basement membrane relative to the closest intact squamous mucosa. The greatest depth of invasion is measured by dropping a plumb line from the horizon. Source: From *AJCC Cancer Staging Manual*, 2017. © Springer Nature.

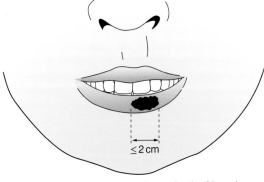

> 5 mm depth of invasion   **Fig. 28**

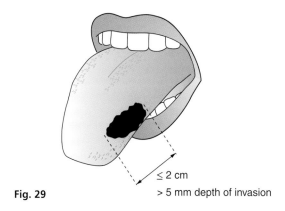

Fig. 29

≤ 2 cm
> 5 mm depth of invasion

T2   pT2

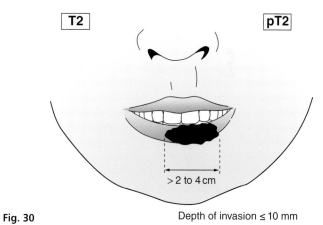

Fig. 30

> 2 to 4 cm

Depth of invasion ≤ 10 mm

T2   pT2

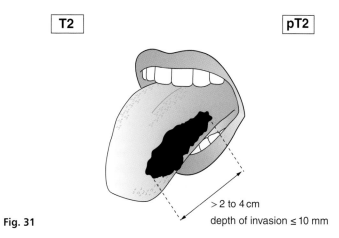

Fig. 31

> 2 to 4 cm
depth of invasion ≤ 10 mm

T3 pT3

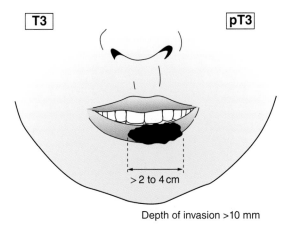

> 2 to 4 cm

Depth of invasion >10 mm   **Fig. 32**

T3 pT3

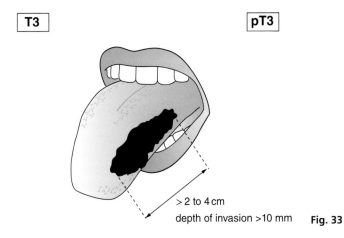

> 2 to 4 cm

depth of invasion >10 mm   **Fig. 33**

T3 pT3

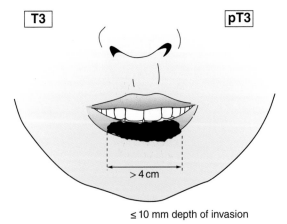

> 4 cm

≤ 10 mm depth of invasion   **Fig. 34**

T3   pT3

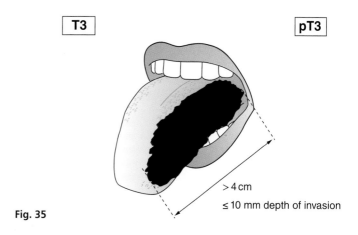

> 4 cm

≤ 10 mm depth of invasion

Fig. 35

T4a   pT4a

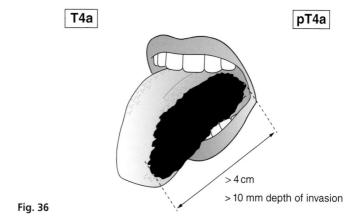

> 4 cm

> 10 mm depth of invasion

Fig. 36

T4a   pT4a

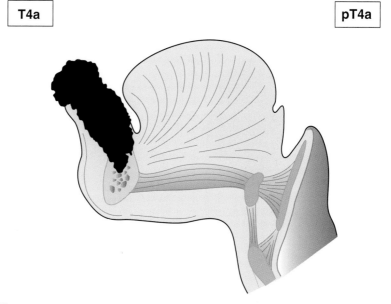

Fig. 37

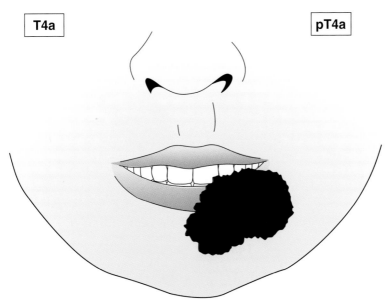

Fig. 38

T4a   Continued
       (Oral Cavity) – Tumour invades through the cortical bone of the mandible or
       maxilla or involves the maxillary sinus, or invades the skin of the face (Fig. 39)

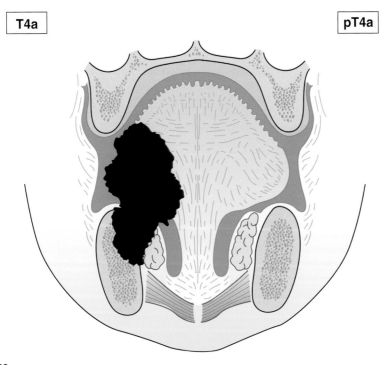

Fig. 39

T4b   *(lip and oral cavity)* Tumour invades masticator space, pterygoid plates or skull base, or encases internal carotid artery (Fig. 40)

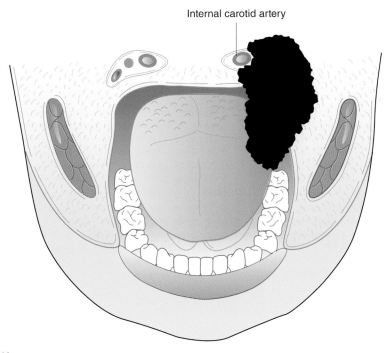

Fig. 40

PHARYNX (ICD-O C01, C05.1, 2, C09, C10.0, 2, 3, C11–13)

Rules for Classification

The classification applies only to carcinomas. There should be histological confirmation of the disease.

Anatomical Sites and Subsites

Oropharynx (C01, C05.1, 2, C09.0, 1, 9, C10.0, 2, 3) (Figs. 41, 42)

1. Anterior wall (glosso-epiglottic area)
   (i) Base of tongue (posterior to the vallate papillae or posterior third) (C01)
   (ii) Vallecula (C10.0)
2. Lateral wall (C10.2)
   (i) Tonsil (C09.9)
   (ii) Tonsillar fossa (C09.0) and tonsillar (faucial) pillars (C09.1)
   (iii) Glossotonsillar sulci (tonsillar pillars) (C09.1)
3. Posterior wall (C10.3)
4. Superior wall
   (i) Inferior surface of soft palate (C05.1)
   (ii) Uvula (C05.2)

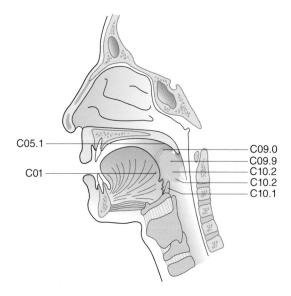

Fig. 41

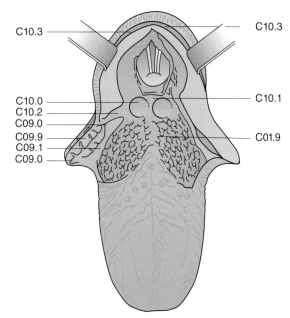

C10.3

C10.3

C10.0
C10.2
C09.0
C09.9
C09.1
C09.0

C10.1

C01.9

Fig. 42

Note
The lingual (anterior) surface of the epiglottis (C10.1) is included with the larynx, suprahyoid epiglottis (see pages 35–36).

Nasopharynx (Fig. 43)

1. Postero-superior wall: extends from the level of the junction of the hard and soft palates to the base of the skull (C11.0, 1)
2. Lateral wall: including the fossa of Rosenmüller (C11.2)
3. Inferior wall: consists of the superior surface of the soft palate (C11.3)

Note
The margin of the choanal orifices, including the posterior margin of the nasal septum, is included with the nasal fossa.

Hypopharynx (C12, C13) (Fig. 43)

1. Pharyngo-oesophageal junction (postcricoid area) (C13.0): extends from the level of the arytenoid cartilages and connecting folds to the inferior border of the cricoid cartilage, thus forming the anterior wall of the hypopharynx
2. Piriform sinus (C12.9): extends from the pharyngoepiglottic fold to the upper end of the oesophagus. It is bounded laterally by the thyroid cartilage and medially by the hypopharyngeal surface of the aryepiglottic fold (C13.1) and the arytenoid and cricoid cartilages
3. Posterior pharyngeal wall (C13.2): extends from the superior level of the hyoid bone (or floor of the vallecula) to the level of the inferior border of the cricoid cartilage and from the apex of one piriform sinus to the other

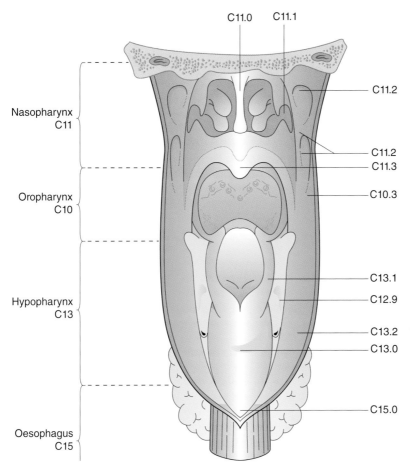

Fig. 43

Regional Lymph Nodes

The regional lymph nodes are the cervical nodes.

The supraclavicular fossa (relevant to classifying nasopharyngeal carcinoma) is the triangular region defined by three points:

1. the superior margin of the sternal end of the clavicle;
2. the superior margin of the lateral end of the clavicle;
3. the point where the neck meets the shoulder. This includes caudal portions of Levels IV and V (classification according to Robbins et al.[2]).

[2] Robbins KT, Median JE, Wolfe GT, Levine PA, Sesions RB, Pruet CW (1991) Standardizing neck dissection terminology. Official report of the Academy's Committee for Head and Neck Surgery and Oncology. *Arch Otolaryngol Head Neck Surg* 117:601–605.

TN Clinical Classification

T – Primary Tumour

TX   Primary tumour cannot be assessed
T0   No evidence of primary tumour
Tis   Carcinoma in situ

Oropharynx

p16 negative cancers of the oropharynx, or oropharyngeal cancers without a p16 immunohistochemistry performed

T1   Tumour 2 cm or less in greatest dimension (Fig. 44)
T2   Tumour more than 2 cm but not more than 4 cm in greatest dimension (Fig. 45)

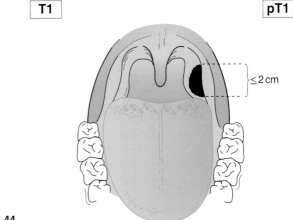

T1   pT1

≤ 2 cm

Fig. 44

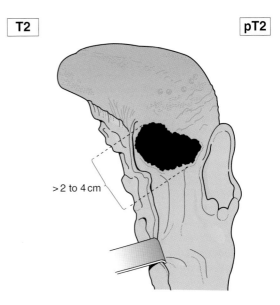

T2   pT2

> 2 to 4 cm

Fig. 45

T3   Tumour more than 4 cm in greatest dimension or extension to lingual surface of epiglottis (Fig. 46)

T4a   Tumour invades any of the following: larynx, deep/extrinsic muscle of tongue (genioglossus, hyoglossus, palatoglossus and styloglossus), medial pterygoid, hard palate or mandible* (Fig. 47)

T4b   Tumour invades any of the following: lateral pterygoid muscle, pterygoid plates, lateral nasopharynx, skull base; or encases carotid artery (Fig. 48)

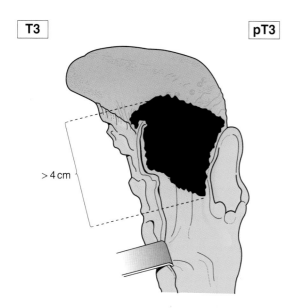

| T3 | pT3 |

> 4 cm

Fig. 46

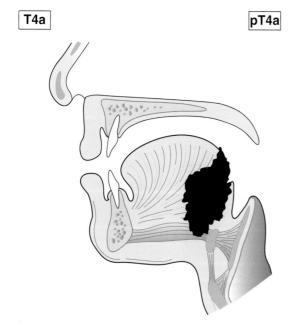

| T4a | pT4a |

Fig. 47

T4b   pT4b

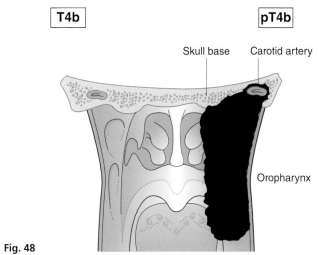

Skull base   Carotid artery

Oropharynx

Fig. 48

Note

*Mucosal extension to lingual surface of epiglottis from primary tumours of the base of the tongue and vallecula does not constitute invasion of the larynx.

Oropharynx – p16-Positive Tumours

Tumours that have positive p16 immunohistochemistry overexpression.

T1   Tumour 2 cm or less in greatest dimension (Fig. 44)
T2   Tumour more than 2 cm but not more than 4 cm in greatest dimension (Fig. 45)
T3   Tumour more than 4 cm in greatest dimension or extension to lingual surface of epiglottis (Fig. 46)
T4   Tumour invades any of the following: larynx, deep/extrinsic muscle of tongue (genioglossus, hyoglossus, palatoglossus and styloglossus), medial pterygoid, hard palate, mandible*, lateral pterygoid muscle, pterygoid plates, lateral nasopharynx, skull base; or encases carotid artery (Figs. 47, 48, 49)

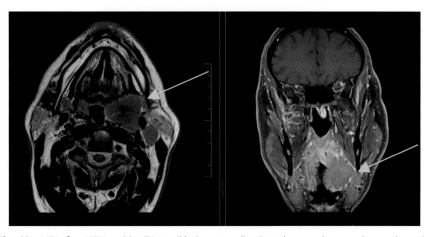

Fig. 49   MRI of an HPV-positive T4 tonsil lesion extending into the parapharyngeal space (arrow).

Nasopharynx

T1 Tumour confined to nasopharynx, or extends to oropharynx and/or nasal cavity (Fig. 50)

T2 Tumour with extension to parapharyngeal space and/or infiltration of the medial pterygoid, lateral pterygoid and/or prevertebral muscles (Figs. 51, 52)

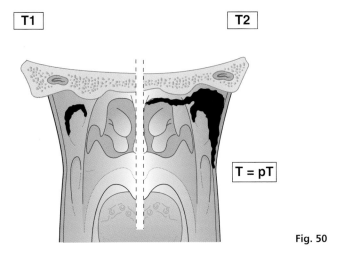

T1   **T2**

T = pT

Fig. 50

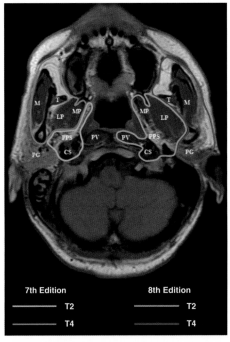

Fig. 51 Differences in defining criteria between the previous 7th edition and the current 8th edition: changing the extent of soft tissue involvement as T2 and T4 criteria. CS indicates carotid space; LP, lateral pterygoid muscle; M, masseter muscle; MP, medial pterygoid muscle; PG, parotid gland; PPS, parapharyngeal space; PV, prevertebral muscle; T, temporalis muscle. Source: Modified from Pan JJ, Ng WT, Zong JF, et al. (2016) Proposal for the 8th edition of the AJCC/UICC staging system for nasopharyngeal cancer in the era of intensity-modulated radiotherapy. *Cancer* 122(4):546–558.

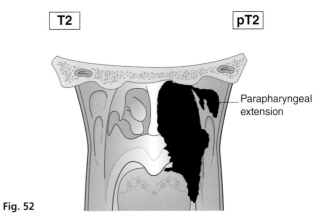

Parapharyngeal extension

Fig. 52

T3   Tumour invades bony structures of skull base cervical vertebra, pterygoid structures and/or paranasal sinuses (Fig. 53)

T4   Tumour with intracranial extension and/or involvement of cranial nerves, hypopharynx, orbit, parotid gland and/or infiltration beyond the lateral surface of the lateral pterygoid muscle (Fig. 54)

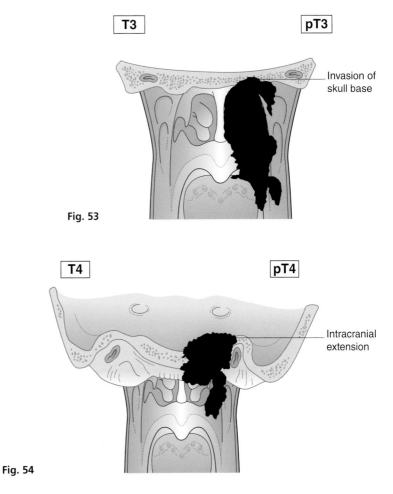

Invasion of skull base

Fig. 53

Intracranial extension

Fig. 54

Hypopharynx

T1   Tumour limited to one subsite of hypopharynx (see Fig. 43) and/or 2 cm or less in greatest dimension (Figs. 55, 56, 57)

T2   Tumour invades more than one subsite of hypopharynx or an adjacent site, or measures more than 2 cm but not more than 4 cm in greatest dimension, without fixation of hemilarynx (Figs. 58, 59, 60, 61, 62)

T3   Tumour more than 4 cm in greatest dimension, or *with* fixation of hemilarynx or extension to oesophagus (Figs. 63, 64, 65)

T4a   Tumour invades any of the following: thyroid/cricoid cartilage, hyoid bone, thyroid gland, oesophagus, central compartment soft tissue* (Figs. 66, 67)

T4b   Tumour invades prevertebral fascia (Fig. 68), encases carotid artery or invades mediastinal structures

Note
*Central compartment soft tissue includes prelaryngeal strap muscles and subcutaneous fat.

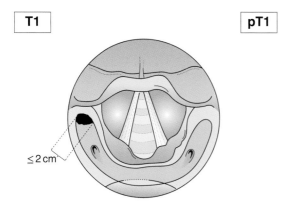

Fig. 55

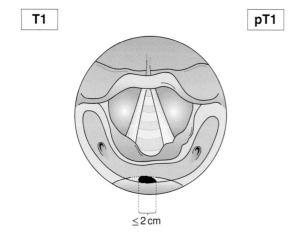

Fig. 56

T1   pT1

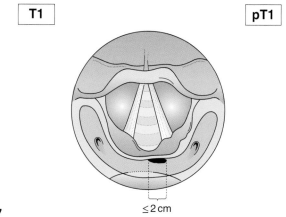

≤ 2 cm

Fig. 57

T2   pT2

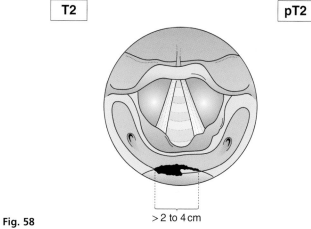

> 2 to 4 cm

Fig. 58

T2   pT2

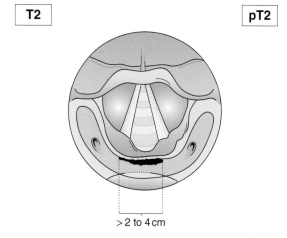

> 2 to 4 cm

Fig. 59

T2   pT2

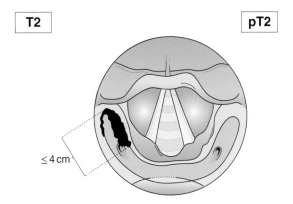

Fig. 60

T2   pT2

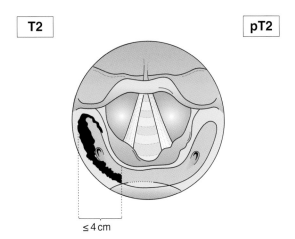

Fig. 61

T2   pT2

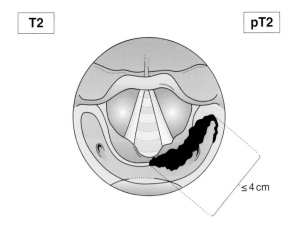

Fig. 62

T3   pT3

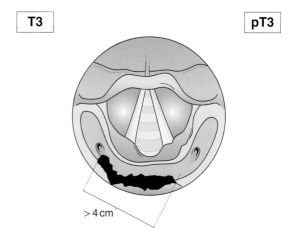

> 4 cm

Fig. 63

T3   pT3

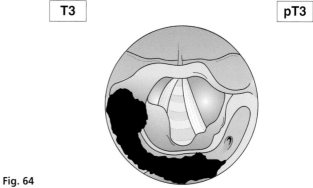

Fig. 64

T3   pT3

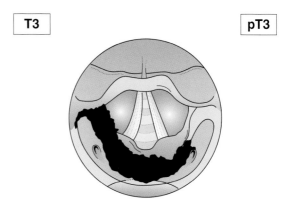

Fig. 65

T4a   pT4a

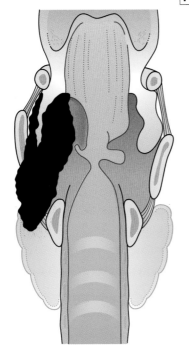

Fig. 66

T4a   pT4a

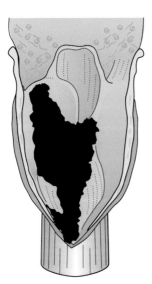

Fig. 67

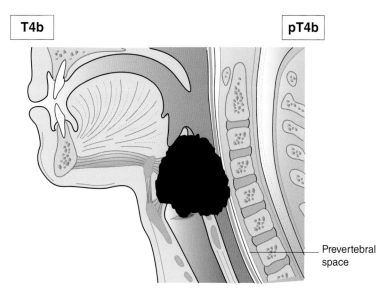

Fig. 68

p16-Negative Oro- and Hypopharynx

N – Regional Lymph Nodes

See Head and Neck Tumours for p16-negative oropharynx tumours and hypopharynx.

p16-Positive Oropharynx

Clinical

NX   Regional lymph nodes cannot be assessed
N0   No regional lymph node metastasis
N1   Unilateral metastasis, in lymph node(s), all 6 cm or less in greatest dimension (Fig. 69)
N2   Contralateral or bilateral metastasis in lymph node(s), all 6 cm or less in greatest dimension (Fig. 70)
N3   Metastasis in lymph node(s) greater than 6 cm in dimension (Fig. 71)

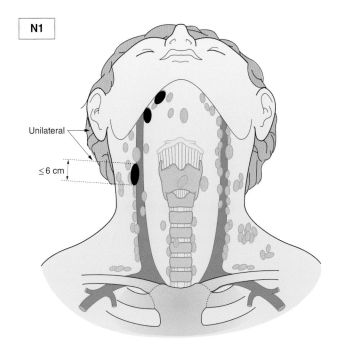

Fig. 69

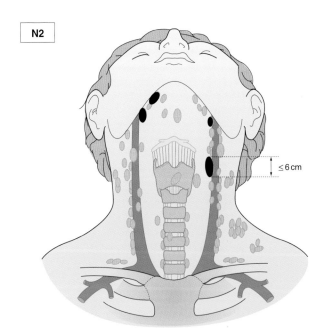

Fig. 70

N3

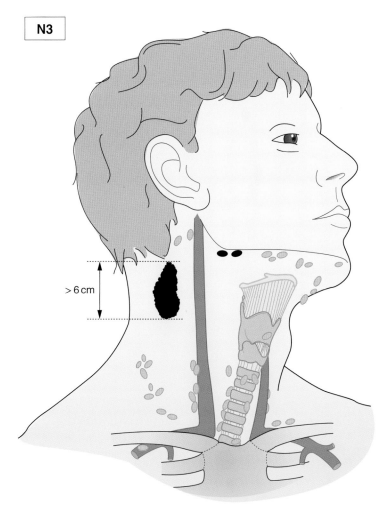

> 6 cm

Fig. 71

Pathological

pNX	Regional lymph nodes cannot be assessed
pN0	No regional lymph node metastasis
pN1	Metastasis in 1 to 4 lymph node(s) (Fig. 72)
pN2	Metastasis in 5 or more lymph nodes (Fig. 73)

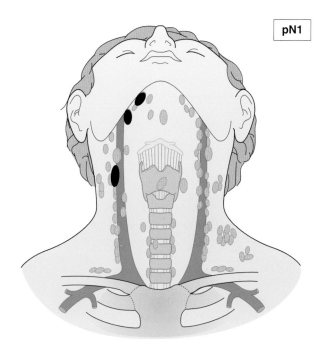

pN1

Fig. 72

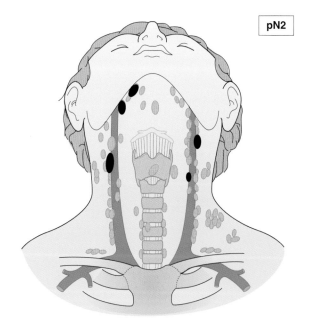

pN2

Fig. 73

Nasopharynx

N – Regional Lymph Nodes

NX   Regional lymph nodes cannot be assessed
N0   No regional lymph node metastasis
N1   Unilateral metastasis, in cervical lymph node(s), and/or unilateral or bilateral metastasis in retropharyngeal lymph nodes, 6 cm or less in greatest dimension, above the caudal border of cricoid cartilage (Fig. 74)
N2   Bilateral metastasis in cervical lymph node(s), 6 cm or less in greatest dimension, above the caudal border of cricoid cartilage (Fig. 75, 76)
N3   Metastasis in cervical lymph node(s) greater than 6 cm in dimension and/or extension below the caudal border of cricoid cartilage (Fig. 76, 77)

Note
Midline nodes are considered ipsilateral nodes.

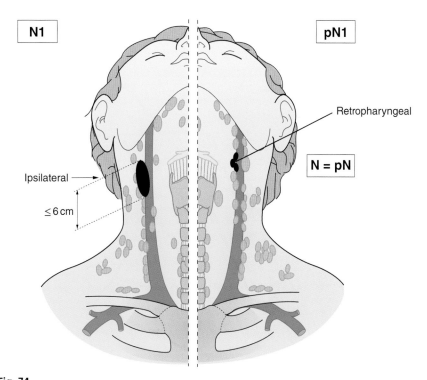

Fig. 74

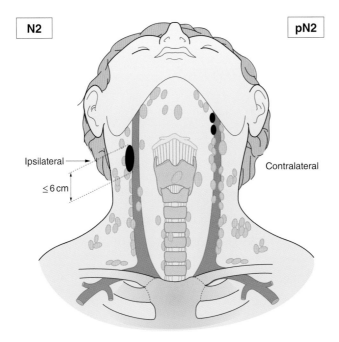

Fig. 75

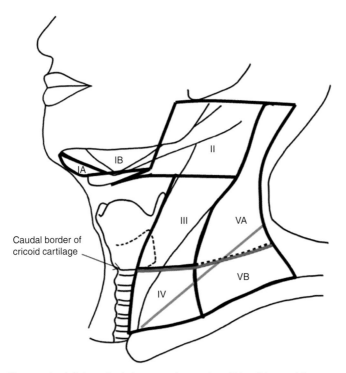

Fig. 76   Differences in defining criteria between the previous 7th edition and the current 8th edition: replacing the supraclavicular fossa (blue) with the lower neck (i.e., below the caudal border of cricoid cartilage; red) as N3 criteria. Source: Modified from Pan JJ, Ng WT, Zong JF, et al. (2016) Proposal for the 8th edition of the AJCC/UICC staging system for nasopharyngeal cancer in the era of intensity-modulated radiotherapy. *Cancer* 122(4):546–558.

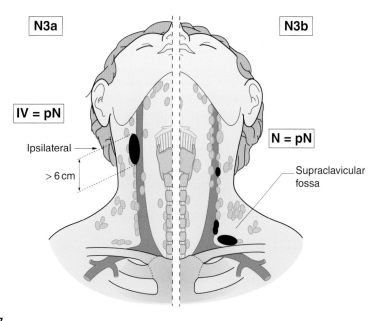

Fig. 77

pTN Pathological Classification

The pT and pN categories correspond to the T and N categories.

Summary

Pharynx	
Oropharynx p16 negative	
T1	≤ 2 cm
T2	> 2 to 4 cm
T3	> 4 cm
T4a	Larynx, deep/extrinsic muscle of tongue, medial pterygoid, hard palate, mandible
T4b	Lateral pterygoid muscle, pterygoid plates, lateral nasopharynx, skull base, carotid artery
Oropharynx p16 positive	
T1	≤ 2 cm
T2	> 2 to 4 cm
T3	> 4 cm
T4	Larynx, deep muscles, of tongue, lateral pterygoid muscle, bone or encases carotid
Hypopharynx	
T1	≤ 2 cm and limited to one subsite
T2	> 2 to 4 cm or more than one subsite
T3	> 4 cm or with hemilarynx fixation

(continued)

Pharynx (*continued*)

T4a	Thyroid/cricoid cartilage, hyoid bone, thyroid gland, oesophagus, central compartment soft tissue
T4b	Prevertebral fascia, carotid artery, mediastinal structures

Nasopharynx

T1	Nasopharynx, oropharynx or nasal cavity
T2	Parapharyngeal extension
T3	Bony structures of skull base/paranasal sinuses
T4	Intracranial, cranial nerves, hypopharynx, orbit, infratemporal fossa/masticator space

LARYNX (ICD-O C32.0, 1, 2, C10.1)

The classification applies only to carcinomas. There should be histological confirmation of the disease.

Anatomical Sites and Subsites

(Figs. 41, 42, 78, 79)

1. Supraglottis (C32.1)

(i) Suprahyoid epiglottis [including tip, lingual (anterior) (C10.1), and laryngeal surfaces]   *Epilarynx (including marginal zone)*

(ii) Aryepiglottic fold, laryngeal aspect

(iii) Arytenoid

(iv) Infrahyoid epiglottis   *Supraglottis excluding epilarynx*

(v) Ventricular bands (false cords)

2. Glottis (C32.0)

(i) Vocal cords

(ii) Anterior commissure

(iii) Posterior commissure

3. Subglottis (C32.2)

Regional Lymph Nodes

See Head and Neck Tumours.

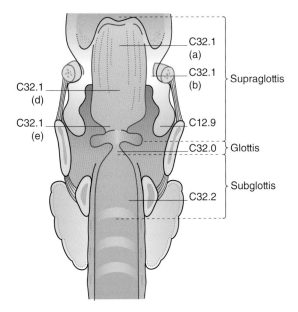

Fig. 78

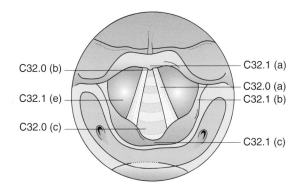

Fig. 79

TNM Clinical Classification

T – Primary Tumour

TX   Primary tumour cannot be assessed
T0   No evidence of primary tumour
Tis   Carcinoma in situ

Supraglottis

T1   Tumour limited to one subsite of supraglottis with normal vocal cord mobility
(Figs. 80, 81)

(a) 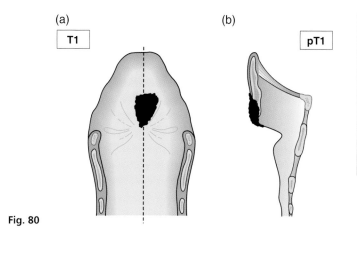 (b)

Fig. 80

(a) 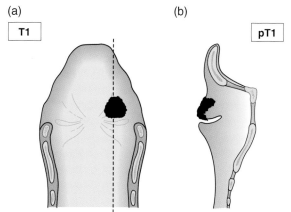 (b)

Fig. 81

T2   Tumour invades mucosa of more than one adjacent subsite of supraglottis or glottis or region outside the supraglottis (e.g., mucosa of base of tongue, vallecula or medial wall of piriform sinus) without fixation of the larynx (Figs. 82, 83)

T3   Tumour limited to larynx with vocal cord fixation and/or invades any of the following: postcricoid area, pre-epiglottic space, paraglottic space and/or inner cortex of thyroid cartilage (Figs. 84, 85)

T4a   Tumour invades through the thyroid cartilage and/or invades tissues beyond the larynx, e.g., trachea, soft tissues of neck including deep/extrinsic muscle of tongue (genioglossus, hyoglossus, palatoglossus and styloglossus), strap muscles, thyroid, oesophagus (Fig. 86)

T4b   Tumour invades prevertebral space, mediastinal structures, or encases carotid artery (Fig. 68)

(a)

T2

(b)

pT2

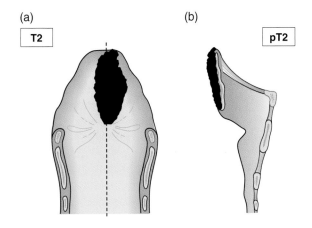

Fig. 82

(a)

T2

(b)

T2

T = pT

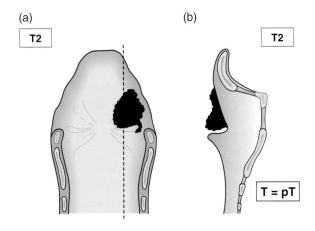

Fig. 83

(a)

T3

(b)

T3

T = pT

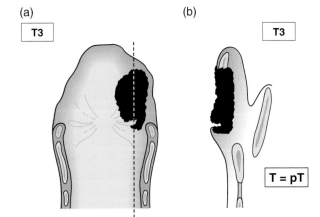

Fig. 84

(a)   (b)

T3   T3

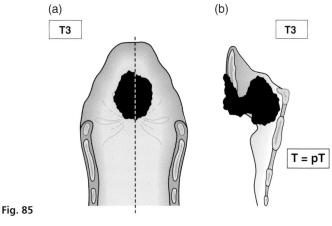

T = pT

Fig. 85

(a)   (b)

T4a   T4a

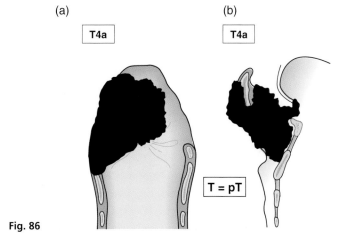

T = pT

Fig. 86

Glottis

T1   Tumour limited to vocal cord(s) (may involve anterior or posterior commissure) with normal mobility (Fig. 87a)

T1a   Tumour limited to one vocal cord (Fig. 87b)

T1b   Tumour involves both vocal cords (Fig. 87c)

T2   Tumour extends to supraglottis and/or subglottis, and/or with impaired vocal cord mobility (Fig. 88)

T3   Tumour limited to larynx with vocal cord fixation and/or invades paraglottic space, and/or inner cortex of the thyroid cartilage (Fig. 89)

T4a   Tumour invades through the outer cortex of the thyroid cartilage, and/or invades tissues beyond the larynx, e.g., trachea, soft tissues of neck including deep/extrinsic muscle of tongue (genioglossus, hyoglossus, palatoglossus and styloglossus), strap muscles, thyroid, oesophagus (Fig. 90)

T4b   Tumour invades prevertebral space, encases carotid artery, or mediastinal structures (Fig. 91)

(a)

T1   pT1

(b)

T1a   pT1a

(c)

T1b   pT1b

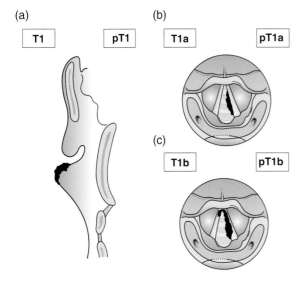

Fig. 87

(a)

T2

(b)

T2

T = pT

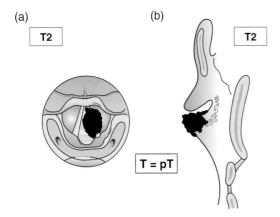

Fig. 88

(a)

T3

(b)

T3

T = pT

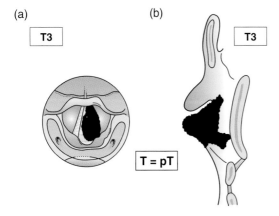

Fig. 89

(a)   (b)

T4a   T4a

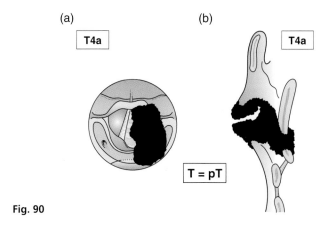

T = pT

Fig. 90

T4b

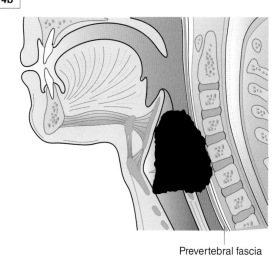

Fig. 91   Prevertebral fascia

Subglottis

T1   Tumour limited to subglottis (Fig. 92)

T2   Tumour extends to vocal cord(s) with normal or impaired mobility (Fig. 93)

T3   Tumour limited to larynx with vocal cord fixation (Fig. 94)

T4a   Tumour invades cricoid or thyroid cartilage and/or invades tissues beyond the larynx, e.g., trachea, soft tissues of neck including deep/extrinsic muscle of tongue (genioglossus, hyoglossus, palatoglossus and styloglossus), strap muscles, thyroid, oesophagus (Fig. 95)

T4b   Tumour invades prevertebral space, mediastinal structures, or encases carotid artery (Fig. 96)

(a)

(b)

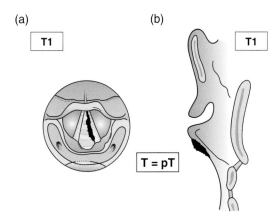

T1

T1

T = pT

Fig. 92

(a)

(b)

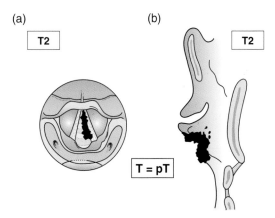

T2

T2

T = pT

Fig. 93

(a)

(b)

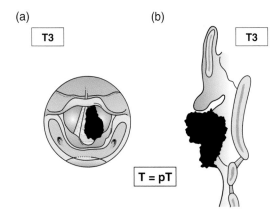

T3

T3

T = pT

Fig. 94

(a)   (b)

T4a

T4a

T = pT

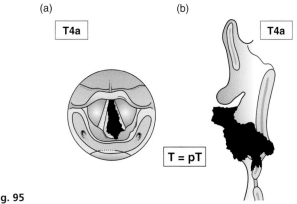

Fig. 95

T4b

pT4b

Prevertebral
fascia

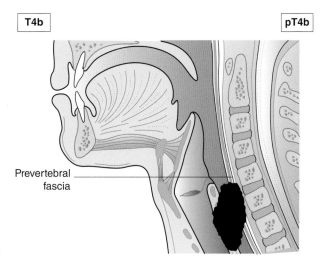

Fig. 96

N – Regional Lymph Nodes

See Head and Neck Tumours.

pTN Pathological Classification

The pT and pN categories correspond to the T and N categories.

Summary

Larynx	
Supraglottis	
T1	One subsite, normal mobility
T2	Mucosa of more than one adjacent subsite of supraglottis or glottis or adjacent region outside the supraglottis; without fixation
T3	Cord fixation or invades postcricoid area, pre-epiglottic tissues, paraglottic space, thyroid cartilage erosion
T4a	Through thyroid cartilage; trachea, soft tissues of neck: deep/extrinsic muscle of tongue, strap muscles, thyroid, oesophagus
T4b	Prevertebral space, mediastinal structures, carotid artery
Glottis	
T1	Limited to vocal cord(s), normal mobility
	(a) one cord
	(b) both cords
T2	Supraglottis, subglottis, impaired cord mobility
T3	Cord fixation, paraglottic space, thyroid cartilage erosion
T4a	Through thyroid cartilage; trachea, soft tissues of neck: deep/extrinsic muscle of tongue, strap muscles, thyroid, oesophagus
T4b	Prevertebral space, mediastinal structures, carotid artery
Subglottis	
T1	Limited to subglottis
T2	Extends to vocal cord(s) with normal/impaired mobility
T3	Cord fixation
T4a	Through cricoid or thyroid cartilage; trachea, deep/extrinsic muscle of tongue, strap muscles, thyroid, oesophagus
T4b	Prevertebral space, mediastinal structures, carotid artery

NASAL CAVITY AND PARANASAL SINUSES (ICD-O C30.0, 31.0, 1)

Rules for Classification

The classification applies only to carcinomas. There should be histological confirmation of the disease.

Anatomical Sites and Subsites

1. *Nasal Cavity (C30.0) (Fig. 97)*
   – Septum
   – Floor
   – Lateral wall
   – Vestibule

2. *Maxillary Sinus (C31.0) (Fig. 98)*

3. *Ethmoid Sinus (C31.0) (Fig. 98)*
   – Left
   – Right

Regional Lymph Nodes

See Head and Neck Tumours.

TN Clinical Classification

T – Primary Tumour

TX   Primary tumour cannot be assessed
T0   No evidence of primary tumour
Tis   Carcinoma in situ

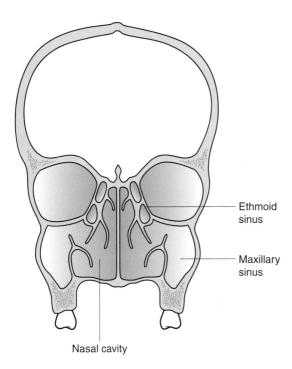

Ethmoid sinus

Maxillary sinus

Nasal cavity

Fig. 97

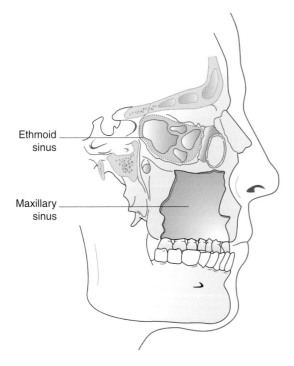

Ethmoid sinus

Maxillary sinus

Fig. 98

Maxillary Sinus

T1   Tumour limited to the mucosa with no erosion or destruction of bone (Fig. 99)

T2   Tumour causing bone erosion or destruction, including extension into the hard palate and/or middle nasal meatus, except extension to posterior wall of maxillary sinus and pterygoid plates (Fig. 100)

T3   Tumour invades any of the following: bone of posterior wall of maxillary sinus, subcutaneous tissues, floor or medial wall of orbit, pterygoid fossa, ethmoid sinuses (Figs. 101, 102)

T4a   Tumour invades any of the following: anterior orbital contents, skin of cheek, pterygoid plates, infratemporal fossa, cribriform plate, sphenoid or frontal sinuses (Figs. 103, 104)

T4b   Tumour invades any of the following: orbital apex, dura, brain, middle cranial fossa, cranial nerves other than maxillary division of trigeminal nerve (V2), nasopharynx or clivus (Fig. 105)

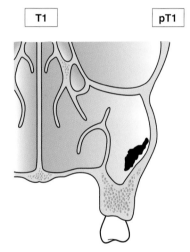

T1   pT1

Fig. 99

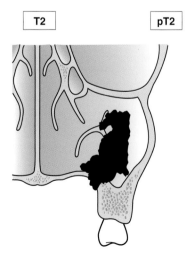

T2   pT2

Fig. 100

T3   T3

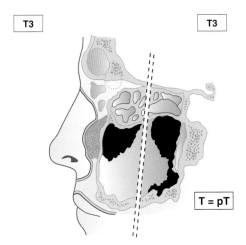

T = pT

Fig. 101

T3   T3

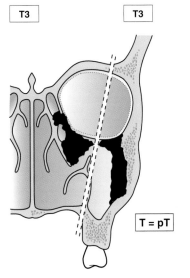

T = pT

Fig. 102

T4a   pT4a

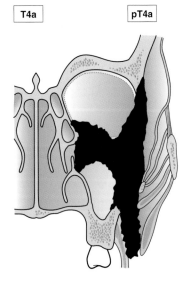

Fig. 103

T4a   pT4a

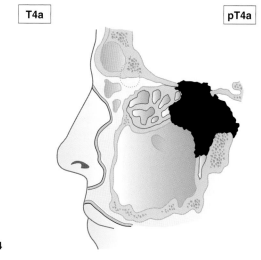

Fig. 104

T4b   pT4b

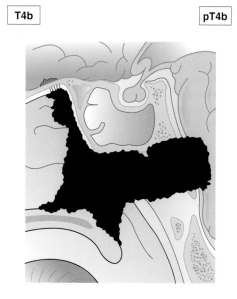

Fig. 105

Nasal Cavity and Ethmoid Sinus

T1   Tumour restricted to one subsite of nasal cavity or ethmoid sinus, with or without bony invasion (Figs. 106, 107)

T2   Tumour involves two subsites in a single site or extends to involve an adjacent site within the nasoethmoidal complex, with or without bony invasion (Fig. 108)

T3   Tumour extends to invade the medial wall or floor of the orbit, maxillary sinus, palate, or cribriform plate (Fig. 109)

T4a   Tumour invades any of the following: anterior orbital contents, skin of nose or cheek, minimal extension to anterior cranial fossa, pterygoid plates, sphenoid or frontal sinuses (Fig. 110)

T4b   Tumour invades any of the following: orbital apex, dura, brain, middle cranial fossa, cranial nerves other than V2, nasopharynx or clivus (Fig. 111)

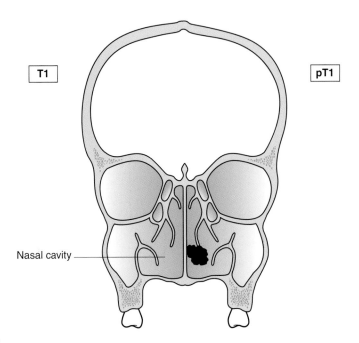

Fig. 106

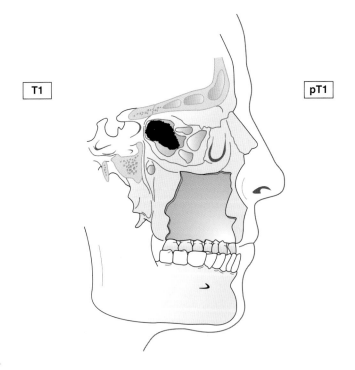

Fig. 107

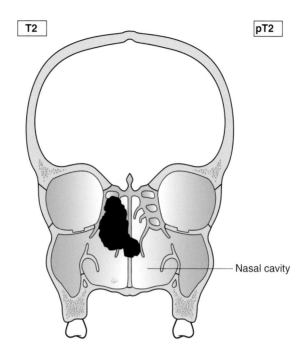

Fig. 108

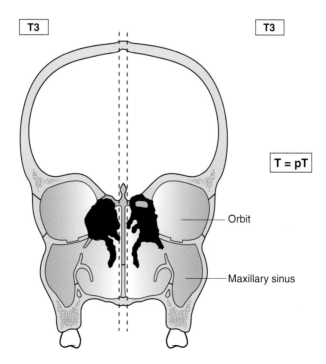

Fig. 109

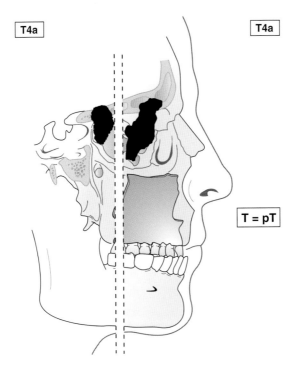

Fig. 110

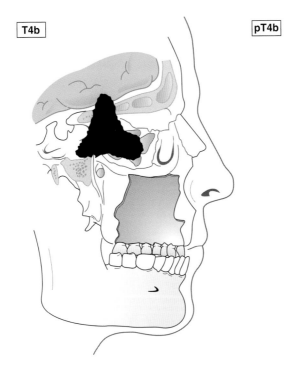

Fig. 111

Regional Lymph Nodes

See Head and Neck Tumours.

pTN Pathological Classification

The pT and pN categories correspond to the T and N categories.

Summary

Nasal Cavity and Paranasal Sinuses	
Maxillary Sinus	
T1	Mucosa
T2	Bone erosion/destruction, hard palate, middle nasal meatus
T3	Posterior bony wall maxillary sinus, subcutaneous tissues, floor/medial wall of orbit, pterygoid fossa, ethmoid sinus
T4a	Anterior orbit, cheek skin, pterygoid plates, infratemporal fossa, cribriform plate, sphenoid/frontal sinus
T4b	Orbital apex, dura, brain, middle cranial fossa, cranial nerves other than V2, nasopharynx, clivus
Nasal Cavity and Ethmoid Sinus	
T1	One subsite
T2	Two subsites or adjacent nasoethmoidal site
T3	Medial wall/floor orbit, maxillary sinus, palate, cribriform plate
T4a	Anterior orbit, skin of nose/cheek, anterior cranial fossa (minimal), pterygoid plates, sphenoid/frontal sinuses
T4b	Orbital apex, dura, brain, middle cranial fossa, cranial nerves other than V2, nasopharynx, clivus

UNKNOWN PRIMARY – CERVICAL NODES

Rules for Classification

There should be histological confirmation of squamous cell carcinoma with lymph node metastases, but without an identified primary carcinoma. Histological methods should be used to identify EBV and HPV/p16-related tumours. If there is evidence of EBV, the Nasopharyngeal Classification is applied. If there is evidence of HPV and positive immunohistochemistry p16 overexpression, the p16-positive Oropharyngeal Classification is applied.

TNM Clinical Classification: EBV or HPV/p16 negative or unknown

T – Primary Tumour

T0   No evidence of primary tumour

N – Regional Lymph Nodes

N1   Metastasis in a single lymph node, 3 cm or less in greatest dimension without extranodal extension (Fig. 4)

N2   Metastasis as described below:

    N2a   Metastasis in a single lymph node, more than 3 cm but not more than 6 cm in greatest dimension without extranodal extension (Fig. 5)

    N2b   Metastasis in multiple ipsilateral lymph nodes, none more than 6 cm in greatest dimension without extranodal extension (Fig. 6)

    N2c   Metastasis in bilateral lymph nodes, none more than 6 cm in greatest dimension without extranodal extension (Fig. 7)

N3a   Metastasis in a lymph node more than 6 cm in greatest dimension without extranodal extension (Fig. 8)

N3b   Metastasis in a single or multiple lymph nodes with clinical extranodal extension* (Fig. 9, 10)

Note

* The presence of skin involvement or soft tissue invasion with deep fixation/tethering to underlying muscle or adjacent structures or clinical signs of nerve involvement is classified as clinical extranodal extension.

   Midline nodes are considered ipsilateral nodes.

M – Distant Metastasis

M0   No distant metastasis
M1   Distant metastasis

pTNM Pathological Classification

There is no pT category. For pM, see pages XX.

pN – Regional Lymph Nodes

Histological examination of a selective neck dissection specimen will ordinarily include 10 or more lymph nodes. Histological examination of a radical or modified radical neck dissection specimen will ordinarily include 15 or more lymph nodes.

pN1   Metastasis in a single lymph node, 3 cm or less in greatest dimension without extranodal extension (Fig. 11)

pN2   Metastasis as described below:

   pN2a   Metastasis in a single lymph node, 3 cm or less in greatest dimension with extranodal extension (Fig. 12) or,
   More than 3 cm but not more than 6 cm in greatest dimension without extranodal extension (Fig. 13)

   pN2b   Metastasis in multiple ipsilateral lymph nodes, none more than 6 cm in greatest dimension without extranodal extension (Fig. 14)

   pN2c   Metastasis in bilateral lymph nodes, none more than 6 cm in greatest dimension without extranodal extension (Fig. 15)

pN3a   Metastasis in a lymph node more than 6 cm in greatest dimension without extranodal extension (Fig. 16)

pN3b   Metastasis in a lymph node more than 3 cm in greatest dimension with extranodal extension or,
   Multiple ipsilateral, or any contralateral, or bilateral node(s), with extranodal extension (Figs. 17, 18)

TNM Clinical Classification – HPV/p16 Positive

T – Primary Tumour

T0   No evidence of primary tumour

N – Regional Lymph Nodes

N1   Unilateral metastasis, in cervical lymph node(s), all 6 cm or less in greatest dimension (Fig. 69)

N2   Contralateral or bilateral metastasis in cervical lymph node(s), all 6 cm or less in greatest dimension (Fig. 70)

N3   Metastasis in cervical lymph node(s) greater than 6 cm in dimension (Fig. 71)

pTNM Pathological Classification

There is no pT category.

  Histological examination of a selective neck dissection specimen will ordinarily include 10 or more lymph nodes.

pN – Regional Lymph Nodes

Histological examination of a radical or modified radical neck dissection specimen will ordinarily include 15 or more lymph nodes.

N – Regional Lymph Nodes

pN1   Metastasis in 1 to 4 lymph node(s) (Fig. 72)

pN2   Metastasis in 5 or more lymph nodes (Fig. 73)

TNM Clinical Classification – EBV positive

T – Primary Tumour

T0   No evidence of primary tumour

N – Regional Lymph Nodes *(Nasopharynx)*

N1 Unilateral metastasis, in cervical lymph node(s), and/or unilateral or bilateral metastasis in retropharyngeal lymph nodes, 6 cm or less in greatest dimension, above the caudal border of cricoid cartilage (Fig. 74)

N2 Bilateral metastasis in cervical lymph node(s), 6 cm or less in greatest dimension, above the caudal border of cricoid cartilage (Figs. 75, 76)

N3 Metastasis in cervical lymph node(s) greater than 6 cm in dimension and/or extension below the caudal border of cricoid cartilage (Figs. 76, 77)

Note
Midline nodes are considered ipsilateral nodes.

pTNM Pathological Classification

There is no pT category. The pN categories correspond to the N categories. For pM see page XX.

pN0 Histological examination of a selective neck dissection specimen will ordinarily include 10 or more lymph nodes. Histological examination of a radical or modified radical neck dissection specimen will ordinarily include 15 or more lymph nodes. If the lymph nodes are negative, but the number ordinarily examined is not met, classify as pN0. When size is a criterion for pN classification, measurement is made of the metastasis, not of the entire lymph node.

M – Distant Metastasis

M0 No distant metastasis
M1 Distant metastasis

MALIGNANT MELANOMA OF UPPER AERODIGESTIVE TRACT (ICD-O C00–06,10–14, 30–32)

Rules for Classification

The classification applies only to mucosal malignant melanomas of the head and neck region, i.e., of the upper aerodigestive tract. There should be histological confirmation of the disease and division of cases by site.

Regional Lymph Nodes

The regional lymph nodes are those appropriate to the site of the primary tumour. See Head and Neck Tumours.

TN Clinical Classification

T – Primary Tumour

TX   Primary tumour cannot be assessed
T0   No evidence of primary tumour
T3   Tumour limited to the epithelium and/or submucosa (mucosal disease) (Fig. 112)
T4a   Tumour invades deep soft tissue, cartilage, bone or overlying skin (Fig. 113)
T4b   Tumour invades any of the following: brain, dura, skull base, lower cranial nerves (IX, X, XI, XII), masticator space, carotid artery, prevertebral space, mediastinal structures (Fig. 114)

Note
Mucosal melanomas are aggressive tumours, therefore T1 and T2 are omitted, as are stages I and II (Figs. 113, 114)

(a)

T3

pT3

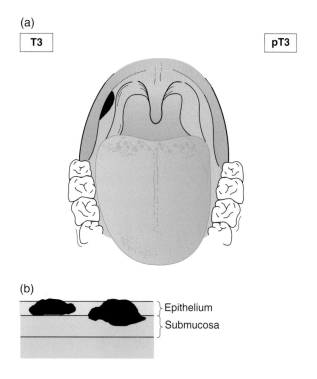

(b)

Epithelium

Submucosa

Fig. 112

T4a

pT4a

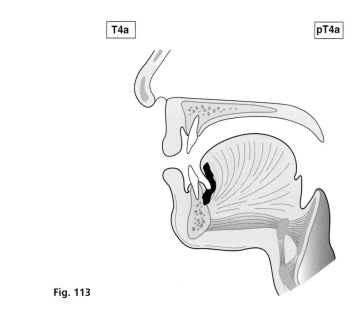

Fig. 113

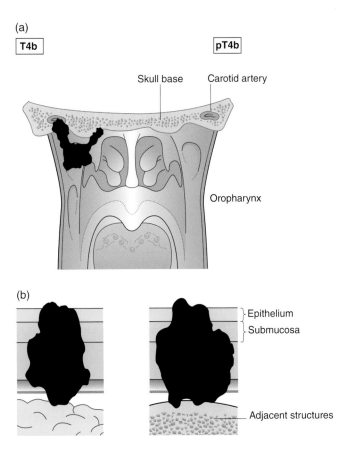

(a)

T4b   pT4b

Skull base   Carotid artery

Oropharynx

(b)

Epithelium
Submucosa

Adjacent structures

Fig. 114

Regional Lymph Nodes

NX   Regional lymph nodes cannot be assessed
N0   No regional lymph node metastasis
N1   Regional lymph node metastasis

pTN Pathological Classification

The pT and pN categories correspond to the T and N categories.

Summary

Melanoma: Upper Aerodigestive Tract
T3   Epithelium/submucosa (mucosal disease)
T4a   Deep soft tissue, cartilage, bone or overlying skin
T4b   Brain, dura, skull base, lower cranial nerves, masticator space, carotid artery, prevertebral space, mediastinal structures

MAJOR SALIVARY GLANDS (ICD-O C07, C08)

Rules for Classification

The classification applies only to carcinomas of the major salivary glands. Tumours arising in minor salivary glands (mucus-secreting glands in the lining membrane of the upper aerodigestive tract) are not included in this classification but at their anatomical site of origin, e.g., the lip. There should be histological confirmation of the disease.

Anatomical Sites

- Parotid gland (C07.9)
- Submandibular (submaxillary) gland (C08.0)
- Sublingual gland (C08.1)

Regional Lymph Nodes

See Head and Neck Tumours.

TN Clinical Classification

T – Primary Tumour

TX   Primary tumour cannot be assessed
T0   No evidence of primary tumour
T1   Tumour 2 cm or less in greatest dimension without extraparenchymal extension* (Fig. 115)
T2   Tumour more than 2 cm but not more than 4 cm in greatest dimension without extraparenchymal extension* (Fig. 116)
T3   Tumour more than 4 cm and/or tumour with extraparenchymal extension* (Figs. 117, 118)
T4a   Tumour invades skin, mandible, ear canal and/or facial nerve (Fig. 119)
T4b   Tumour invades base of skull, and/or pterygoid plates, and/or encases carotid artery (Fig. 120)

Note
*Extraparenchymal extension is clinical or macroscopic evidence of invasion of soft tissues or nerve, except those listed under T4a and 4b. Microscopic evidence alone does not constitute extraparenchymal extension for classification purposes.

T1   pT1

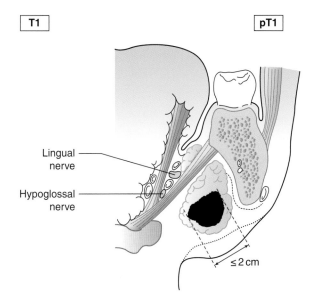

Lingual nerve

Hypoglossal nerve

≤ 2 cm

Fig. 115

T2   pT2

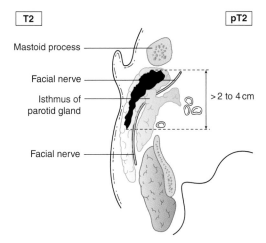

Mastoid process

Facial nerve

Isthmus of parotid gland

Facial nerve

> 2 to 4 cm

Fig. 116

T3   pT3

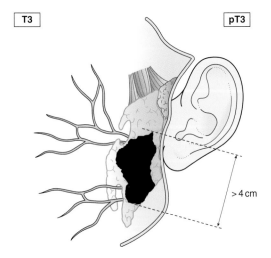

> 4 cm

Fig. 117

T3   pT3

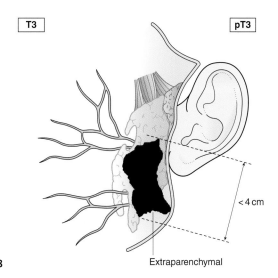

< 4 cm

Extraparenchymal

Fig. 118

T4a   pT4a

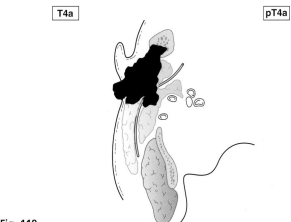

Fig. 119

T4b   pT4b

Skull base

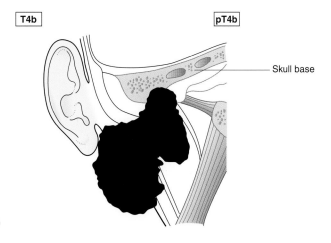

Fig. 120

Regional Lymph Nodes

The regional lymph nodes are the cervical nodes.

pTN Pathological Classification

The pT and pN categories correspond to the T and N categories.

Summary

Salivary Glands

T1	≤ 2 cm, without extraparenchymal extension
T2	> 2 to 4 cm, without extraparenchymal extension
T3	> 4 cm and/or extraparenchymal extension
T4a	Skin, mandible, ear canal, facial nerve
T4b	Skull, pterygoid plates, carotid artery

THYROID GLAND (ICD-O C73) (FIG. 121)

Rules for Classification

The classification applies only to carcinomas, including papillary, follicular, poorly differentiated, insular, anaplastic and medullary carcinomas. There should be microscopic confirmation of the disease and division of cases by histological type.

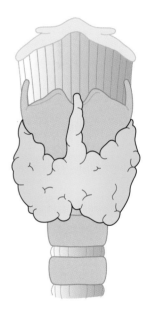

Fig. 121

Regional Lymph Nodes (Fig. 122)

The regional lymph nodes are the cervical and upper/superior mediastinal nodes

TN Clinical Classification

T – Primary Tumour

TX   Primary tumour cannot be assessed
T0   No evidence of primary tumour
T1   Tumour 2 cm or less in greatest dimension, limited to the thyroid (Fig. 123)
     T1a   Tumour 1 cm or less in greatest dimension, minimal extrathyroidal extension may be present

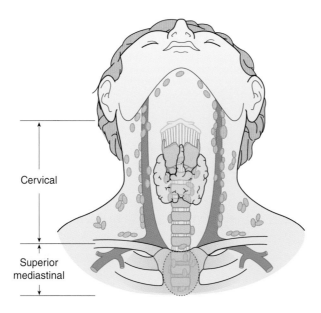

Fig. 122

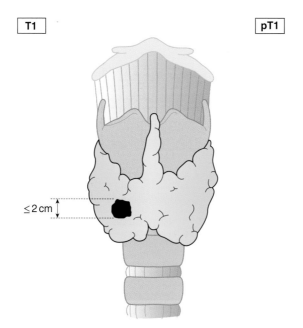

Fig. 123

T1b   Tumour more than 1 cm but not more than 2 cm in greatest dimension, minimal extrathyroidal extension may be present

T2   Tumour more than 2 cm but not more than 4 cm in greatest dimension, minimal extrathyroidal extension may be present (Fig. 124, 125)

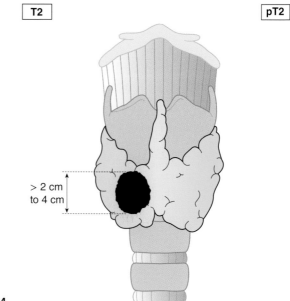

Fig. 124

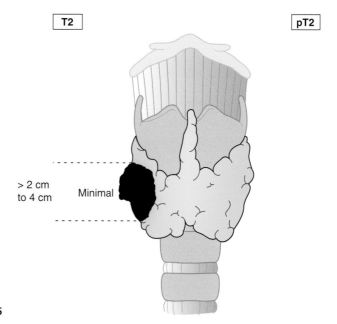

Fig. 125

T3a   Tumour more than 4 cm in greatest dimension, limited to the thyroid or with minimal extrathyroid extension (Fig. 126)

T3b   Tumour of any size with gross extrathyroid extension invading the strap muscles (e.g., extension to sternohyoid, sternothyroid or omohyoid muscles)

T3

pT3

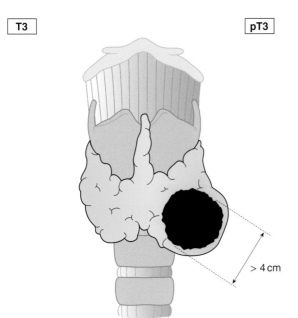

> 4 cm

Fig. 126

T4a   Tumour extends beyond the thyroid capsule and invades any of the following: subcutaneous soft tissues, larynx, trachea, oesophagus, recurrent laryngeal nerve (Figs. 127, 128)

T4b   Tumour invades prevertebral fascia, mediastinal vessels, or encases carotid artery (Fig. 129)

T4a

pT4a

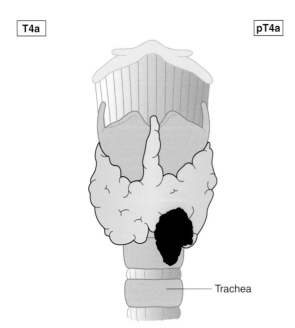

Trachea

Fig. 127

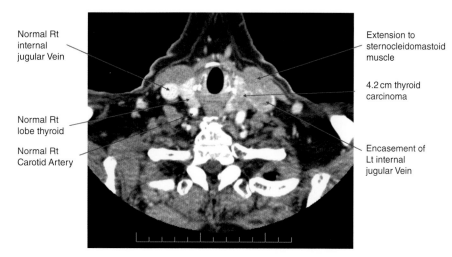

Normal Rt internal jugular Vein

Normal Rt lobe thyroid

Normal Rt Carotid Artery

Extension to sternocleidomastoid muscle

4.2 cm thyroid carcinoma

Encasement of Lt internal jugular Vein

Fig. 128

T4b

pT4b

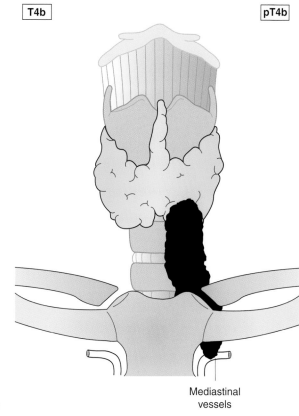

Mediastinal vessels

Fig. 129

N – Regional Lymph Nodes

NX   Regional lymph nodes cannot be assessed

N0   No regional lymph node metastasis

N1   Regional lymph node metastasis

      N1a   Metastasis in Level VI (pretracheal, paratracheal and prelaryngeal/ Delphian lymph nodes) or upper/superior mediastinum (Fig. 130)

      N1b   Metastasis in other unilateral, bilateral or contralateral cervical (Levels I, II, III, IV or V) or retropharyngeal (Fig. 131)

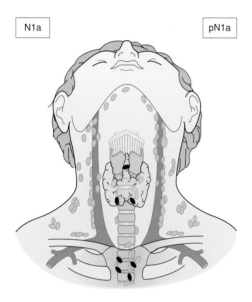

Fig. 130

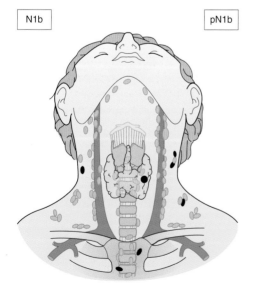

Fig. 131

pTN Pathological Classification

The pT and pN categories correspond to the T and N categories.

Histopathologic Types

The four major histopathologic types are:
- Papillary carcinoma (including those with follicular foci)
- Follicular carcinoma (including so-called Hürthle cell carcinoma)
- Medullary carcinoma
- Anaplastic/undifferentiated carcinoma

Summary

Thyroid Gland	
Papillary, Follicular, Anaplastic and Medullary Carcinoma	
T1	≤ 2 cm
T2	> 2 to 4 cm
T3a	> 4 cm or minimal extension
T3b	Gross extrathyroid extension into strap muscles
T4a	Subcutaneous, larynx, trachea, oesophagus, recurrent laryngeal nerve
T4b	Prevertebral fascia, mediastinal vessels, carotid artery
All Types	
N1a	Level VI
N1b	Other regional

DIGESTIVE SYSTEM TUMOURS

Introductory Notes

The following sites and types are included:
- Oesophagus and oesophagogastric junction
- Stomach
- Small intestine
- Appendix
- Colon and rectum
- Anal canal and perianal skin
- Liver cell carcinoma
- Intrahepatic cholangiocarcinoma
- Gallbladder
- Perihilar bile duct
- Distal extrahepatic bile duct
- Ampulla of Vater
- Pancreas
- Neuroendocrine tumours

Each site is described under the following headings:
- Rules for classification with the procedures for assessing T, N and M categories; additional methods may be used when they enhance the accuracy of appraisal before treatment
- Anatomical sites and subsites where appropriate
- Definition of the regional lymph nodes
- TNM clinical classification
- pTNM pathological classification
- G histopathological grading where appropriate
- Stage

Regional Lymph Nodes

The number of lymph nodes ordinarily included in a lymphadenectomy specimen is noted at each site.

TNM Atlas: Illustrated Guide to the TNM Classification of Malignant Tumours, Seventh Edition.
Edited by James D. Brierley, Hisao Asamura, Elisabeth Van Eycken, and Brian Rous.
© 2021 by UICC. Published 2021 by John Wiley & Sons Ltd.

OESOPHAGUS (ICD-O-3 C15)
INCLUDING OESOPHAGOGASTRIC
JUNCTION (ICD-O-3 C16.0)

The classification applies only to carcinomas and includes adenocarcinomas of the oesophagogastric/gastroesophageal junction. There should be histological confirmation of the disease and division of cases by topographic localization and histological type. A tumour the epicentre of which is within 2 cm of the oesophagogastric junction and also extends into the oesophagus is classified and staged using the oesophageal scheme. Cancers involving the oesophagogastric junction whose epicentre is within the proximal 2 cm of the cardia (Siewert types I/II) are to be staged as oesophageal cancers.

Anatomical Subsites (Figs. 132, 133)

1. Cervical oesophagus (C15.0): this commences at the lower border of the cricoid cartilage and ends at the thoracic inlet (suprasternal notch), approximately 18 cm from the upper incisor teeth.
2. Intrathoracic oesophagus
   (a) The upper thoracic portion (C15.3) extending from the thoracic inlet to the level of the tracheal bifurcation, approximately 24 cm from the upper incisor teeth
   (b) The mid-thoracic portion (C15.4) is the proximal half of the oesophagus between the tracheal bifurcation and the oesophagogastric junction. The lower level is approximately 32 cm from the upper incisor teeth
   (c) The lower thoracic portion (C15.5), approximately 8 cm in length (includes abdominal oesophagus), is the distal half of the oesophagus between the tracheal bifurcation and the oesophagogastric junction. The lower level is approximately 40 cm from the upper incisor teeth
3. Oesophagogastric junction (C16.0). Cancers involving the oesophagogastric junction whose epicentre is within the proximal 2 cm of the cardia (Siewert types I/II) are to be staged as oesophageal cancers. Cancers whose epicentre is more than 2 cm distal from the oesophagogastric junction will be staged using the Stomach Cancer TNM and Stage, even if the oesophagogastric junction is involved.

Regional Lymph Nodes

The regional lymph nodes, irrespective of the site of the primary tumour, are those in the oesophageal drainage area, including coeliac axis nodes and paraesophageal nodes in the neck, but not the supraclavicular nodes.

TNM Clinical Classification

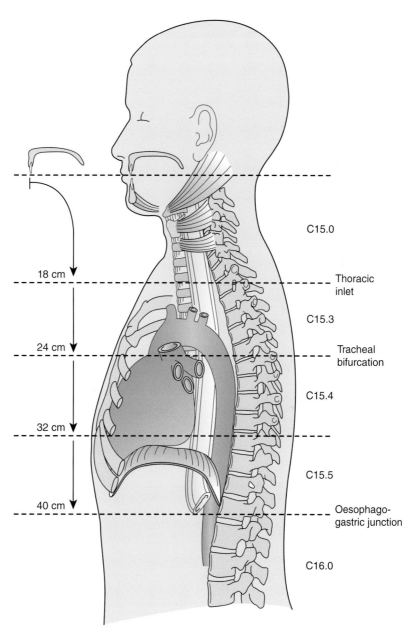

C15.0

18 cm — Thoracic inlet

C15.3

24 cm — Tracheal bifurcation

C15.4

32 cm

C15.5

40 cm — Oesophago-gastric junction

C16.0

Fig. 132

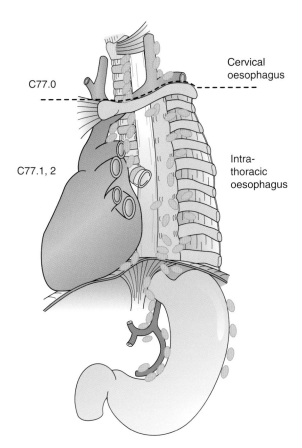

Fig. 133

Regional Lymph Nodes (Fig. 133)

The regional lymph nodes, irrespective of the site of the primary tumour, are those in the oesophageal drainage area, including coeliac axis nodes and paraesophageal nodes in the neck, but not supraclavicular nodes.

TNM Clinical Classification

T – Primary Tumour

TX   Primary tumour cannot be assessed
T0   No evidence of primary tumour
Tis   Carcinoma in situ/high-grade dysplasia
T1   Tumour invades lamina propria, muscularis mucosae or submucosa (Fig. 134)
    T1a   Tumour invades lamina propria or muscularis mucosae
    T1b   Tumour invades submucosa
T2   Tumour invades muscularis propria (Fig. 134)
T3   Tumour invades adventitia (Fig. 135)

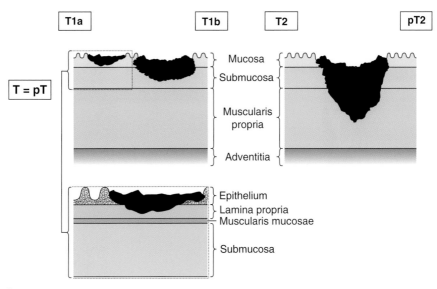

Fig. 134

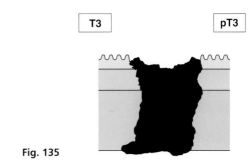

Fig. 135

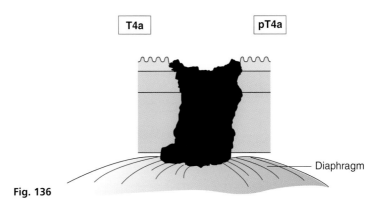

Fig. 136

T4b   pT4b

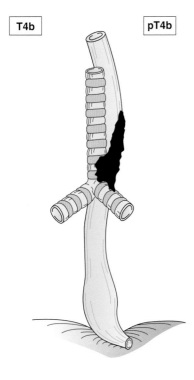

Fig. 137

T4   Tumour invades adjacent structures (Fig. 136)
    T4a   Tumour invades pleura, pericardium, azygos vein, diaphragm or peritoneum
    T4b   Tumour invades other adjacent structures such as aorta, vertebral body or trachea (Fig. 137)

N – Regional Lymph Nodes

NX   Regional lymph nodes cannot be assessed
N0   No regional lymph node metastasis
N1   Metastasis in 1 to 2 regional lymph nodes (Fig. 138)
N2   Metastasis in 3 to 6 regional lymph nodes (Fig. 139)
N3   Metastasis in 7 or more regional lymph nodes (Fig. 140)

M – Distant Metastasis

M0   No distant metastasis
M1   Distant metastasis (Fig. 141)

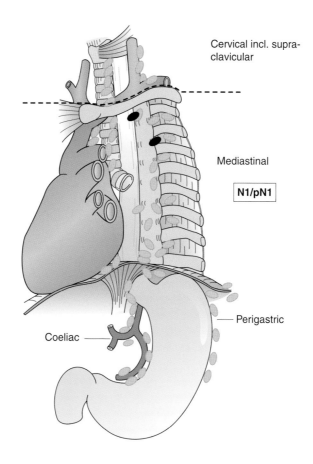

Cervical incl. supra-
clavicular

Mediastinal

N1/pN1

Perigastric

Coeliac

Fig. 138

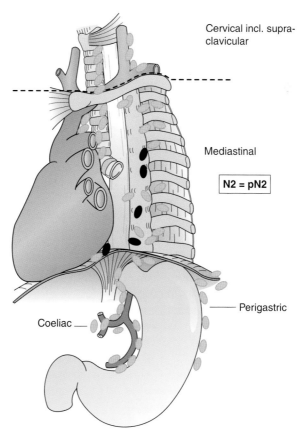

Cervical incl. supra-
clavicular

Mediastinal

N2 = pN2

Perigastric

Coeliac

Fig. 139

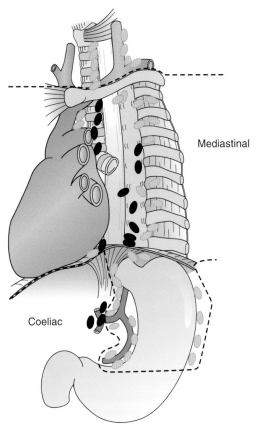

Mediastinal

Coeliac

Fig. 140

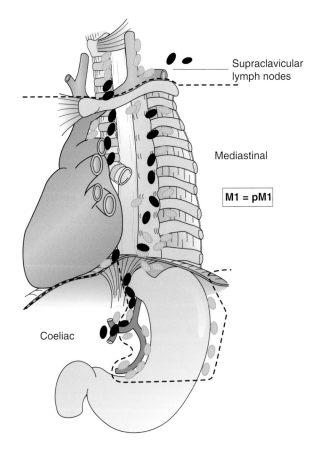

Supraclavicular
lymph nodes

Mediastinal

M1 = pM1

Coeliac

Fig. 141

pTNM Pathological Classification

The pT and pN categories correspond to the T and N categories.

pM1   Distant metastasis microscopically confirmed

Note
pM0 and pMX are not valid categories.

pN0   Histological examination of a regional lymphadenectomy specimen will ordinarily include 6 or more lymph nodes. If the lymph nodes are negative, but the number ordinarily examined is not met, classify as pN0.

Summary

Oesophagus (Includes Oesophagogastric Junction)	
T1	Lamina propria (T1a) submucosa (T1b)
T2	Muscularis propria
T3	Adventitia
T4a	Pleura, pericardium, azygos veil, diaphragm
T4b	Aorta, vertebral body or trachea
N1	1–2 regional
N2	3–6 regional
N3	7 or more regional
M1	Distant metastasis

STOMACH (ICD-O-3 C16)

Rules for Classification

The classification applies only to carcinomas. There should be histological confirmation of the disease. Cancers involving the oesophagogastric junction whose epicentre is within the proximal 2 cm of the cardia (Siewert types I/II) are to be staged as oesophageal cancers. Cancers whose epicentre is more than 2 cm distal from the oesophagogastric junction will be staged using the Stomach Cancer TNM and Stage even if the oesophagogastric junction is involved.

Anatomical Subsites (Fig. 142)

1. Fundus (C16.1)
2. Corpus (C16.2)
3. Antrum (C16.3) and pylorus (C16.4)

Regional Lymph Nodes (Figs. 143, 144)

The regional lymph nodes of the stomach are the perigastric nodes along the lesser (1, 3, 5) and greater (2, 4a, 4b, 6) curvatures, the nodes along the left gastric (7), common hepatic (8), splenic (11) and coeliac arteries (9), and the hepatoduodenal nodes (12).

Involvement of other intra-abdominal lymph nodes such as retropancreatic, mesenteric and para-aortic is classified as distant metastasis.

TNM Clinical Classification

T – Primary Tumour

TX	Primary tumour cannot be assessed
T0	No evidence of primary tumour
Tis	Carcinoma in situ: intraepithelial tumour without invasion of the lamina propria, high-grade dysplasia
T1	Tumour invades lamina propria, muscularis mucosae or submucosa (Fig. 145)
T1a	Tumour invades lamina propria or muscularis mucosae
T1b	Tumour invades submucosa
T2	Tumour invades muscularis propria (Fig. 145)
T3	Tumour invades subserosa (Figs. 145, 146, 147)

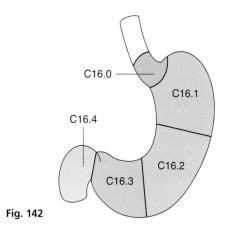

Fig. 142

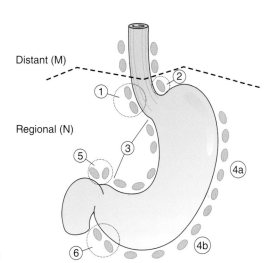

Distant (M)

Regional (N)

Fig. 143

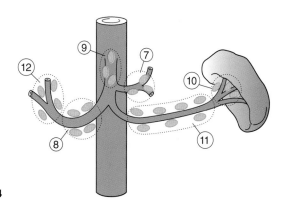

Fig. 144

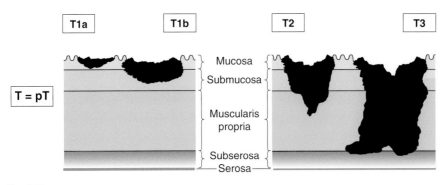

Fig. 145

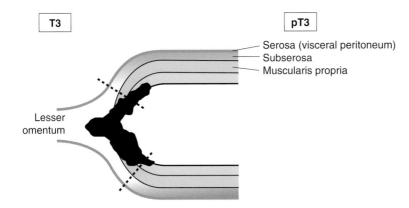

Fig. 146

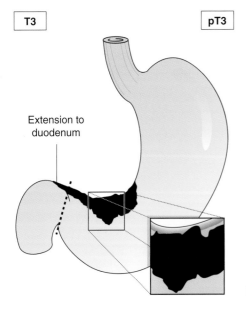

Fig. 147

T4   Tumour perforates serosa (visceral peritoneum) or invades adjacent structures[1,2,3]
    T4a   Tumour perforates serosa
    T4b   Tumour invades adjacent structures[2,3] (Fig. 148)

Notes

[1]The adjacent structures of the stomach are the spleen, transverse colon, liver, diaphragm, pancreas, abdominal wall, adrenal gland, kidney, small intestine and retroperitoneum.

[2]Intramural extension to the duodenum or oesophagus is classified by the depth of greatest invasion in any of these sites including the stomach (Figs. 147, 149).

[3]Tumour that extends into gastrocolic or gastrohepatic ligaments or into greater or lesser omentum, without perforation of visceral peritoneum, is T3 (Fig. 150).

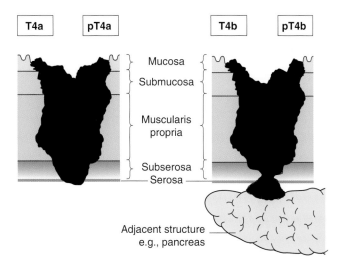

Fig. 148

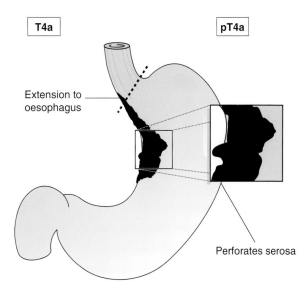

Fig. 149

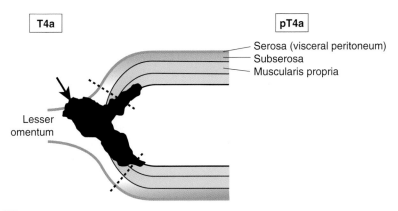

Fig. 150

N – Regional Lymph Nodes

NX   Regional lymph nodes cannot be assessed
N0   No regional lymph node metastasis
N1   Metastasis in 1 to 2 regional lymph nodes (Fig. 151)
N2   Metastasis in 3 to 6 regional lymph nodes (Fig. 152)
N3   Metastasis in 7 or more regional lymph nodes
    N3a   Metastasis in 7 to 15 regional lymph nodes (Fig. 153)
    N3b   Metastasis in 16 or more regional lymph nodes (Fig. 154)

M – Distant Metastasis

M0   No distant metastasis
M1   Distant metastasis (Fig. 154)

Note
Distant metastasis includes peritoneal seeding, positive peritoneal cytology, and omental tumour not part of continuous extension.

pTNM Pathological Classification

The pT and pN categories correspond to the T and N categories.

pM1   Distant metastasis microscopically confirmed
pN0   Histological examination of a regional lymphadenectomy specimen will ordinarily include 16 or more lymph nodes. If the lymph nodes are negative, but the number ordinarily examined is not met, classify as pN0

Note
pM0 and pMX are not valid categories.

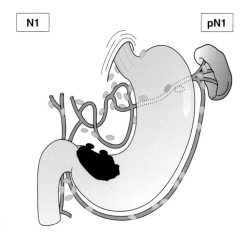

Fig. 151

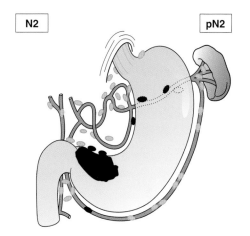

Fig. 152

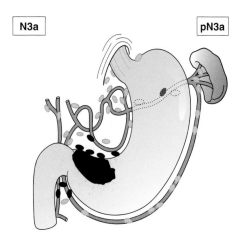

Fig. 153

N3b   pN3b

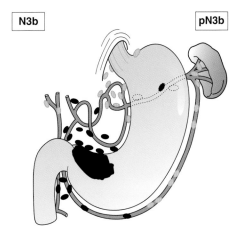

Fig. 154

Summary

Stomach	
T1	Lamina propria (T1a), submucosa (T1b)
T2	Muscularis propria
T3	Subserosa
T4a	Perforates serosa
T4b	Adjacent organs
N1	1–2 regional
N2	3–6 regional
N3a	7–15 regional
N3b	16 or more regional
M1	Distant metastasis

SMALL INTESTINE (ICD-O-3 ICD-O C17)

Rules for Classification

The classification applies only to carcinomas. There should be histological confirmation of the disease.

Anatomical Subsites (Fig. 155)

1. Duodenum (C17.0)
2. Jejunum (C17.1)
3. Ileum (C17.2) (excludes ileocaecal valve C18.0)

Note
This classification does not apply to carcinomas of the ampulla of Vater.

Regional Lymph Nodes

The regional lymph nodes for the duodenum are the pancreaticoduodenal, pyloric, hepatic (pericholedochal, cystic, hilar) and superior mesenteric nodes.

The regional lymph nodes for the ileum and jejunum are the mesenteric nodes, including the superior mesenteric nodes, and, for the terminal ileum only, the ileocolic nodes, including the posterior caecal nodes.

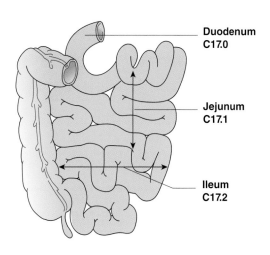

Duodenum
C17.0

Jejunum
C17.1

Ileum
C17.2

Fig. 155

TNM Clinical Classification

T – Primary Tumour

TX   Primary tumour cannot be assessed
T0   No evidence of primary tumour
Tis   Carcinoma in situ
T1   Tumour invades lamina propria, muscularis mucosae or submucosa (Fig. 156)
        T1a   Tumour invades lamina propria or muscularis mucosae
        T1b   Tumour invades submucosa
T2   Tumour invades muscularis propria (Fig. 157)

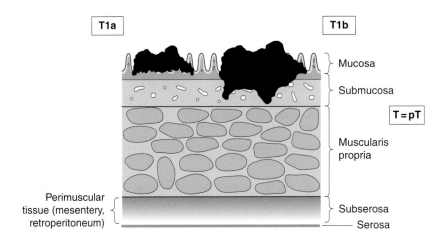

Fig. 156

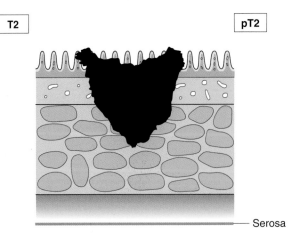

Fig. 157

T3   Tumour invades subserosa or non-peritonealized perimuscular tissue (mesentery or retroperitoneum*) without perforation of the serosa (Fig. 158)

T4   Tumour perforates visceral peritoneum or directly invades other organs or structures (includes other loops of small intestine, mesentery, or retroperitoneum and abdominal wall by way of serosa; for duodenum only, invasion of pancreas) (Figs. 159, 160, 161)

Note

*The non-peritonealized perimuscular tissue is, for jejunum and ileum, part of the mesentery and, for duodenum in areas where serosa is lacking, part of the retroperitoneum.

N – Regional Lymph Nodes

NX   Regional lymph nodes cannot be assessed
N0   No regional lymph node metastasis
N1   Metastasis in 1 to 2 regional lymph nodes
N2   Metastasis in 3 or more regional lymph nodes

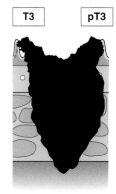

Fig. 158

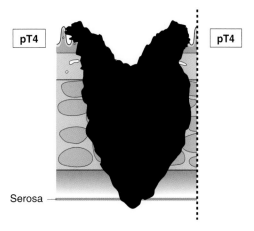

Serosa

Fig. 159

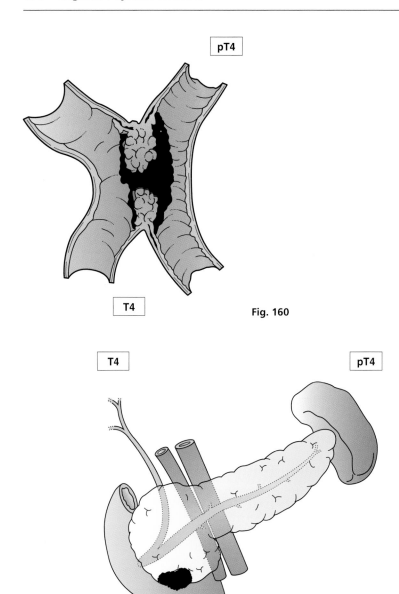

pT4

T4

Fig. 160

T4   pT4

Fig. 161

M – Distant Metastasis

M0   No distant metastasis
M1   Distant metastasis

pTNM Pathological Classification

The pT and pN categories correspond to the T and N categories.

pM1   Distant metastasis microscopically confirmed

Note
pM0 and pMX are not valid categories.

pN0   Histological examination of a regional lymphadenectomy specimen will ordinarily include 6 or more lymph nodes. If the lymph nodes are negative, but the number ordinarily examined is not met, classify as pN0.

Summary

Small Intestine	
T1	Lamina propria, submucosa
T2	Muscularis propria
T3	Subserosa, non-peritonealized perimuscular tissues (mesentery, retroperitoneum)
T4	Visceral peritoneum, other organs/structures
N1	1–2 regional nodes
N2	3 or more regional nodes
M1	Distant metastasis

APPENDIX (ICD-O-3 C18.1)

Rules for Classification

There should be histological confirmation of the disease and separation of carcinomas into mucinous and non-mucinous adenocarcinomas. Goblet cell adenocarcinomas are classified according to the carcinoma scheme. Grading is of particular importance for mucinous tumours.

Anatomical Site

Appendix (C18.1)

Regional Lymph Nodes

The ileocolic are the regional lymph nodes (Fig. 162).

Carcinoma

TNM Clinical Classification

T – Primary Tumour

TX	Primary tumour cannot be assessed
T0	No evidence of primary tumour
Tis	Carcinoma in situ: intraepithelial or invasion of lamina propria[1]
Tis (LAMN)	Low-grade appendiceal mucinous neoplasm confined to the appendix (defined as involvement by acellular mucin or mucinous epithelium that may extend into muscularis propria)
T1	Tumour invades submucosa (Fig. 163)
T2	Tumour invades muscularis propria (Fig. 164)
T3	Tumour invades subserosa or mesoappendix (Fig. 165)
T4	Tumour perforates visceral peritoneum, including mucinous peritoneal tumour within the right lower quadrant and/or directly invades other organs or structures[2,3,4] (Figs. 166, 167)

    T4a   Tumour perforates visceral peritoneum, including mucinous peritoneal tumour within the right lower quadrant (Fig. 166)

    T4b   Tumour directly invades other organs or structures (Figs. 167, 168, 169)

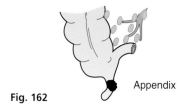

Appendix

Fig. 162

T1 pT1

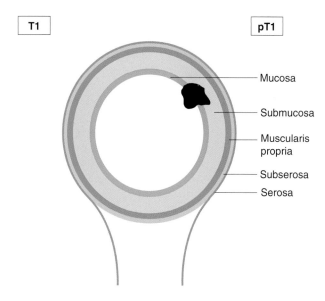

Mucosa

Submucosa

Muscularis propria

Subserosa

Serosa

Fig. 163

T2 pT2

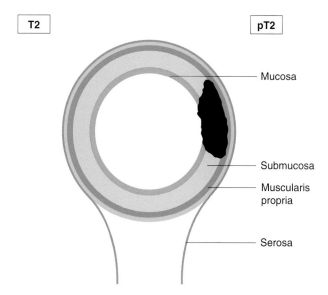

Mucosa

Submucosa

Muscularis propria

Serosa

Fig. 164

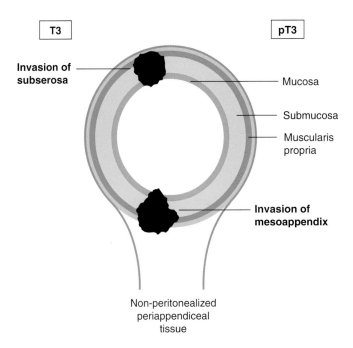

T3   pT3

Invasion of
subserosa

Mucosa

Submucosa

Muscularis
propria

Invasion of
mesoappendix

Non-peritonealized
periappendiceal
tissue

Fig. 165

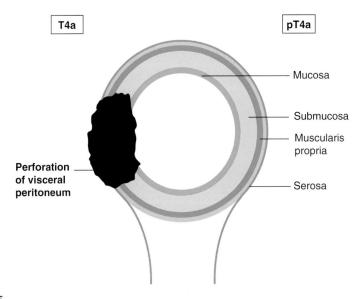

T4a   pT4a

Mucosa

Submucosa

Muscularis
propria

Perforation
of visceral
peritoneum

Serosa

Fig. 166

Notes

[1]Tis includes cancer cells confined within the glandular basement membrane (intraepithelial) or lamina propria (intramucosal) with no extension through muscularis mucosae into submucosa.

[2]Direct invasion in T4 includes invasion of other intestinal segments by way of the serosa, e.g., invasion of ileum.

[3]Tumour that is adherent to other organs or structures, macroscopically, is classified as T4b. However, if no tumour is present in the adhesion, microscopically, the classification should be pT1–3.

[4]LAMN with involvement of the subserosa or the serosal surface should be classified as T3 or T4a respectively.

N – Regional Lymph Nodes

NX   Regional lymph nodes cannot be assessed
N0   No regional lymph node metastasis
N1   Metastasis in 1 to 3 regional lymph nodes (Fig. 168)
    N1a   Metastases in 1 regional lymph node
    N1b   Metastases in 2 to 3 regional lymph nodes
    N1c   Tumour deposit(s), i.e. satellites,* in the subserosa, or in non-peritonealized pericolic or perirectal soft tissue *without* regional lymph node metastasis

N2   Metastasis in 4 or more regional lymph nodes (Fig. 169)

Note

*Tumour deposits (satellites) are discrete macroscopic or microscopic nodules of cancer in the pericolorectal adipose tissue's lymph drainage area of a primary carcinoma that are discontinuous from the primary and without histological evidence of residual lymph node or identifiable vascular or neural structures. If a vessel wall is identifiable on H&E, elastic or other stains, it should be classified as venous invasion (V1/2) or lymphatic invasion (L1). Similarly, if neural structures are identifiable, the lesion should be classified as perineural invasion (Pn1).

M – Distant Metastasis

M0   No distant metastasis
M1   Distant metastasis
    M1a   Intraperitoneal acellular mucin only
    M1b   Intraperitoneal metastasis only
    M1c   Non-peritoneal metastasis

pTNM Pathological Classification

The pT and pN categories correspond to the T and N categories.

pM1   Distant metastasis microscopically confirmed

Note

pM0 and pMX are not valid categories.

pN0   Histological examination of a regional lymphadenectomy specimen will ordinarily include 12 or more lymph nodes. If the lymph nodes are negative, but the number ordinarily examined is not met, classify as pN0.

T4b pT4b

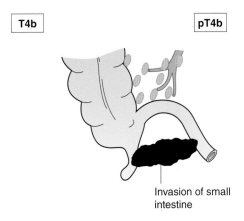

Invasion of small
intestine

Fig. 167

N1 pN1

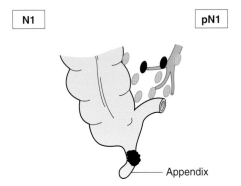

Appendix

Fig. 168

N2 pN2

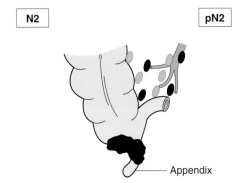

Appendix

Fig. 169

Digestive System

Summary

Appendix Carcinoma

T1	Submucosa
T2	Muscularis propria
T3	Subserosa, non-peritonealized periappendiceal tissues, mesoappendix
T4a	Perforates visceral peritoneum/mucinous peritoneal tumour within right lower quadrant
T4b	Other organs or structures
N1	≤ 3 regional
N2	> 3 regional
M1a	Intraperitoneal acellular mucin only
M1b	Intraperitoneal metastasis only
M1c	Non-peritoneal metastasis

COLON AND RECTUM (ICD-O-3 C18–20)

Rules for Classification

The classification applies only to carcinomas. There should be histological confirmation of the disease.

Anatomical Sites and Subsites

Colon (C18) (Fig. 170)

1. Caecum (C18.0)
2. Ascending colon (C18.2)
3. Hepatic flexure (C18.3)
4. Transverse colon (C18.4)
5. Splenic flexure (C18.5)
6. Descending colon (C18.6)
7. Sigmoid colon (C18.7)

Rectosigmoid junction (C19) (Fig. 171)

Rectum (C20) (Fig. 171)

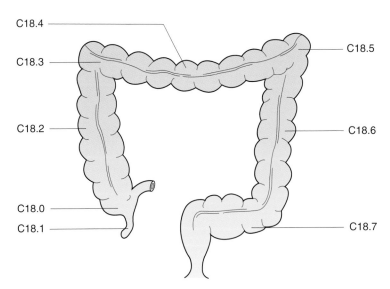

Fig. 170

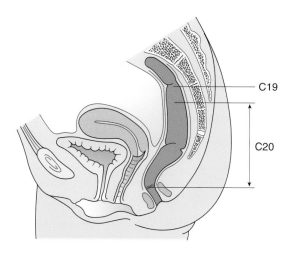

Fig. 171

Regional Lymph Nodes

For each anatomical site or subsite, the following are regional lymph nodes:

Caecum	Ileocolic, right colic (Fig. 172)
Ascending colon	Ileocolic, right colic, middle colic (Fig. 173)
Hepatic flexure	Middle colic, right colic (Fig. 174)
Transverse colon	Right colic, middle colic, left colic, inferior mesenteric (Fig. 175)

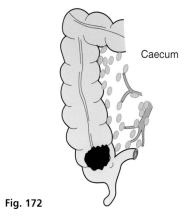

Caecum

Fig. 172

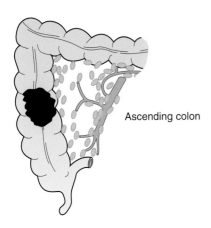

Ascending colon

Fig. 173

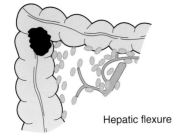

Hepatic flexure   **Fig. 174**

Transverse colon

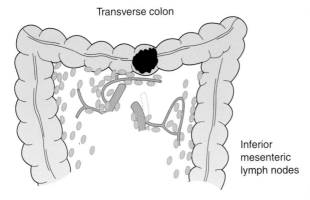

Inferior
mesenteric
lymph nodes

Fig. 175

Splenic flexure	Middle colic, left colic, inferior mesenteric (Fig. 176)
Descending colon	Left colic, inferior mesenteric (Fig. 177)
Sigmoid colon	Sigmoid, left colic, superior rectal (haemorrhoidal), inferior mesenteric and rectosigmoid (Fig. 178)
Rectum	Superior, middle, and inferior rectal (haemorrhoidal), inferior mesenteric, internal iliac, mesorectal (paraproctal), lateral sacral, presacral, sacral promontory (Gerota) (Fig. 179)

Metastasis in nodes other than those listed above is classified as distant metastasis.

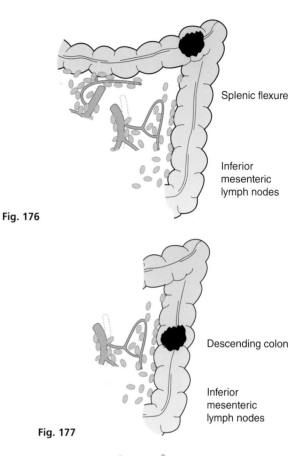

Splenic flexure

Inferior
mesenteric
lymph nodes

Fig. 176

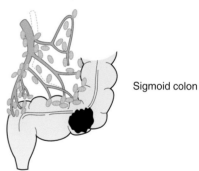

Descending colon

Inferior
mesenteric
lymph nodes

Fig. 177

Sigmoid colon

Fig. 178

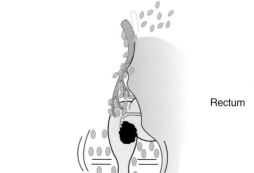

Rectum

Fig. 179

TNM Clinical Classification

T – Primary Tumour

TX   Primary tumour cannot be assessed

T0   No evidence of primary tumour

Tis   Carcinoma in situ: intraepithelial or invasion of lamina propria[1]

T1   Tumour invades submucosa (Fig. 180)

T2   Tumour invades muscularis propria (Fig. 181)

T3   Tumour invades subserosa or into non-peritonealized pericolic or perirectal tissues (Fig. 182)

T4   Tumour directly invades other organs or structures[2,3,4] and/or perforates visceral peritoneum (Figs. 183, 184)

T4a   Tumour perforates visceral peritoneum

T4b   Tumour directly invades other organs or structures

Notes

[1]Tis includes cancer cells confined within mucosal lamina propria (intramucosal) with no extension through the muscularis mucosae into the submucosa.

[2]Invades through to visceral peritoneum to involve the surface.

[3]Direct invasion in T4b includes invasion of other organs or segments of the colorectum by way of the serosa, as confirmed on microscopic examination, or for tumours in a retroperitoneal or subperitoneal location, direct invasion of other organs or structures by virtue of extension beyond the muscularis propria.

[4]Tumour that is adherent to other organs or structures, macroscopically, is classified as cT4b. However, if no tumour is present in the adhesion, microscopically, the classification should be pT1–3, depending on the anatomical depth of wall invasion.

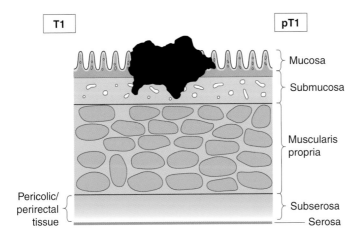

Fig. 180

T2   pT2

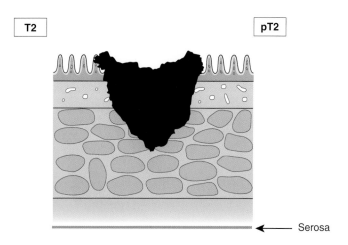

← Serosa

Fig. 181

T3   pT3

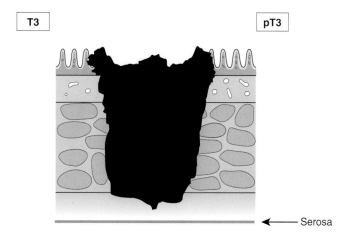

← Serosa

Fig. 182

T4a   pT4a

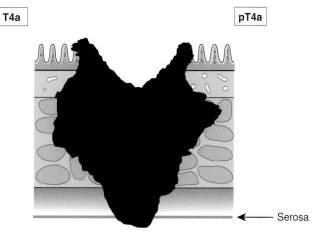

← Serosa

Fig. 183

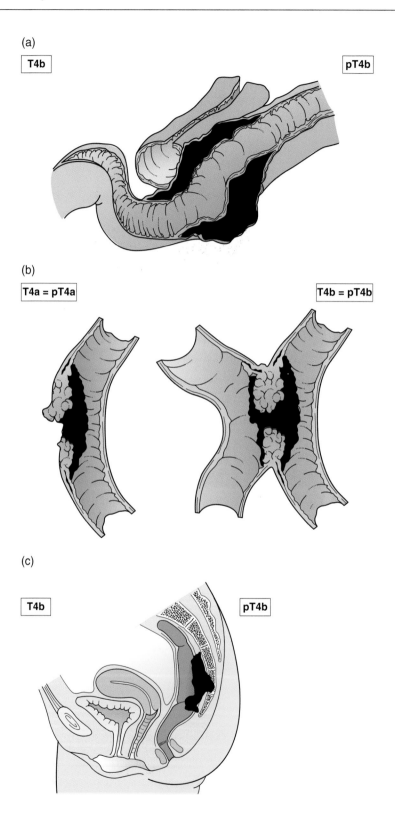

Fig. 184

N – Regional Lymph Nodes

NX   Regional lymph nodes cannot be assessed
N0   No regional lymph node metastasis
N1   Metastasis in 1 to 3 regional lymph nodes (Fig. 185)
    N1a   Metastasis in 1 regional lymph node
    N1b   Metastasis in 2 to 3 regional lymph nodes
    N1c   Tumour deposit(s), i. e. satellites*, in the subserosa, or in non-peritonealized pericolic or perirectal soft tissue *without* regional lymph node metastasis
N2   Metastasis in 4 or more regional lymph nodes (Figs. 186, 187, 188)
    N2a   Metastasis in 4 to 6 regional lymph nodes
    N2b   Metastasis in 7 or more regional lymph nodes

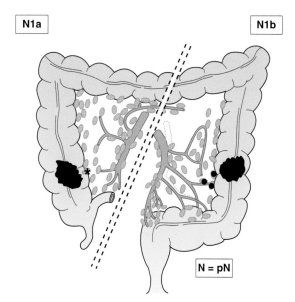

Fig. 185

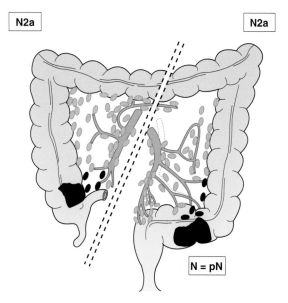

Fig. 186

N2b

N2b

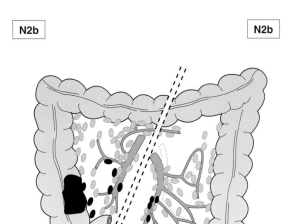

N = pN

Fig. 187

N2b

pN2b

Ligature

Apical node

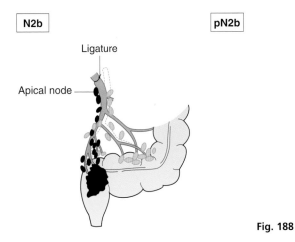

Fig. 188

Note

*Tumour deposits (satellites) are discrete macroscopic or microscopic nodules of cancer in the pericolorectal adipose tissue's lymph drainage area of a primary carcinoma that are discontinuous from the primary and without histological evidence of residual lymph node or identifiable vascular or neural structures. If a vessel wall is identifiable on H&E, elastic or other stains, it should be classified as venous invasion (V1/2) or lymphatic invasion (L1). Similarly, if neural structures are identifiable, the lesion should be classified as perineural invasion (Pn1). The presence of tumour deposits does not change the primary tumour T category, but changes the node status (N) to pN1c if all regional lymph nodes are negative on pathological examination.

M – Distant Metastasis

M0   No distant metastasis
M1   Distant metastasis
    M1a   Metastasis confined to one organ (liver, lung, ovary, non-regional lymph node(s)), without metastases to the peritoneum
    M1b   Metastases in more than one organ without metastases to the peritoneum
    M1c   To peritoneum with or without other organs

TNM Pathological Classification

The pT and pN categories correspond to the T and N categories.

pM1   Distant metastasis microscopically confirmed

Note
pM0 and pMX are not valid categories.

pN0   Histological examination of a regional lymphadenectomy specimen will ordinarily include 12 or more lymph nodes. If the lymph nodes are negative, but the number ordinarily examined is not met, classify as pN0.

Summary

Colon and Rectum	
T1	Submucosa
T2	Muscularis propria
T3	Subserosa, pericolorectal tissues
T4a	Visceral peritoneum
T4b	Other organs or structures
N1a	1 regional
N1b	2–3 regional
N1c	Satellite(s) without regional nodes
N2a	4–6 regional
N2b	7 or more regional
M1a	One organ
M1b	> one organ, peritoneum
M1c	To peritoneum with or without other organs

ANAL CANAL (ICD-O-3 C21, ICD-O-3 C44.5)

The anal canal (Fig. 189) extends from rectum to perianal skin (to the junction with hair-bearing skin). It is lined by the mucous membrane overlying the internal sphincter, including the transitional epithelium and dentate line. Tumours of anal margin and perianal skin defined as within 5 cm of the anal margin (ICD-O-3 C44.5) are now classified with carcinomas of the anal canal (Fig. 190).

Rules for Classification

The classification applies only to carcinomas. There should be histological confirmation of the disease and division of cases by histological type.

Regional Lymph Nodes (Fig. 191)

The regional lymph nodes are the perirectal (1), internal iliac (2), external iliac (3) and inguinal lymph nodes (4).

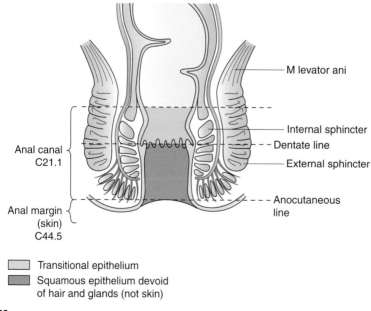

M levator ani

Internal sphincter
Dentate line
External sphincter

Anocutaneous line

Anal canal
C21.1

Anal margin (skin)
C44.5

▢ Transitional epithelium
▨ Squamous epithelium devoid of hair and glands (not skin)

Fig. 189

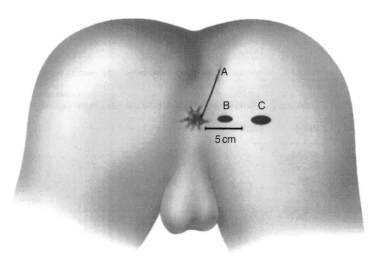

Fig. 190   Source: From Zinner MI, Ashley SW (2012) *Maingot's Abdominal Operations*, 12th edition, McGraw Hill Education. © 2012 McGraw Hill Education.

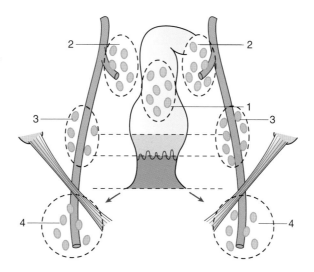

Fig. 191

TNM3 Clinical Classification

T0   No evidence of primary tumour

Tis   Carcinoma in situ, Bowen disease, high-grade squamous intraepithelial neoplasia (HSIL), anal intraepithelial neoplasia (AIN II–III)

T1   Tumour 2 cm or less in greatest dimension (Fig. 192)

T2   Tumour more than 2 but not more than 5 cm in greatest dimension (Fig. 193)

T3   Tumour of more than 5 cm in greatest dimension (Fig. 194)

T4   Tumour of any size invades adjacent organ(s), e.g., vagina, urethra, bladder* (Fig. 195)

T1

pT1

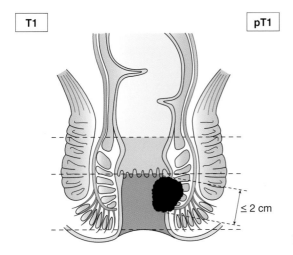

≤ 2 cm

Fig. 192

T2

T2

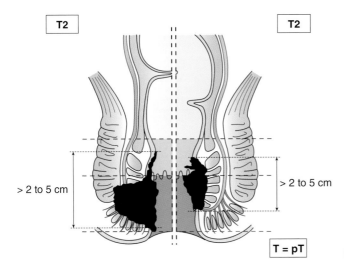

> 2 to 5 cm

> 2 to 5 cm

T = pT

Fig. 193

T3

pT3

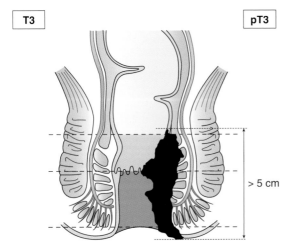

> 5 cm

Fig. 194

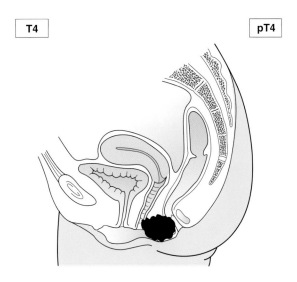

T4   pT4

Fig. 195

Note

*Direct invasion of the rectal wall, perianal skin, subcutaneous tissue or the sphincter muscle(s) *alone* is not classified as T4.

N – Regional Lymph Nodes

NX   Regional lymph nodes cannot be assessed
N0   No regional lymph node metastasis
N1a   Metastases in inguinal, mesorectal and/or internal iliac nodes (Fig. 196)
N1b   Metastases in external iliac nodes (Fig. 197)
N1c   Metastases in external iliac and in inguinal, mesorectal and/or internal iliac nodes (Fig. 198)

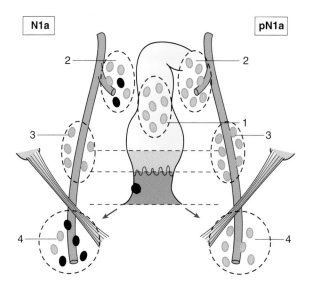

Fig. 196

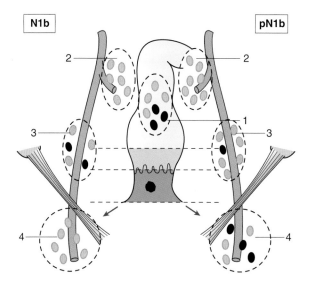

Fig. 197

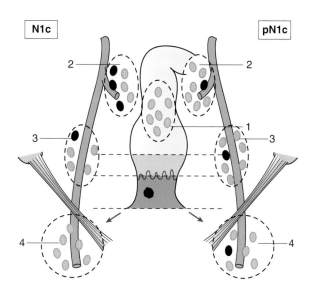

Fig. 198

M – Distant Metastasis

M0   No distant metastasis
M1   Distant metastasis

TNM Pathological Classification

The pT and pN categories correspond to the T and N categories.

pM1   Distant metastasis microscopically confirmed

Note
pM0 and pMX are not valid categories.

pN0   Histological examination of a regional perirectal/pelvic lymphadenectomy specimen will ordinarily include 12 or more lymph nodes; histological examination of an inguinal lymphadenectomy specimen will ordinarily include 6 or more lymph nodes. If the lymph nodes are negative, but the number ordinarily examined is not met, classify as pN0.

Summary

Anal Canal	
T1	≤ 2 cm
T2	> 2 to 5 cm
T3	> 5 cm
T4	Adjacent organs
N1a	Inguinal, mesorectal and/or internal iliac nodes
N1b	External iliac nodes
N1c	External iliac and unguinal, mesorectal and/or internal iliac

LIVER – HEPATOCELLULAR CARCINOMA (ICD-O-3 C22.0)

Rules for Classification

The classification applies only to hepatocellular carcinoma.

Cholangio- (intrahepatic bile duct) carcinoma of the liver has a separate classification (see Liver – Intrahepatic Bile Ducts). There should be histological confirmation of the disease.

Note
Although the presence of cirrhosis is an important prognostic factor, it does not affect the TNM classification, being an independent prognostic variable.

Regional Lymph Nodes (Fig. 199)

The regional lymph nodes are the hilar, hepatic (along the proper hepatic artery), periportal (along the portal vein), inferior phrenic and caval nodes.

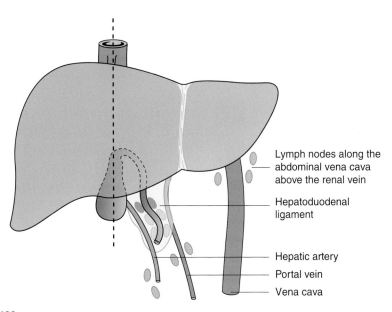

Lymph nodes along the abdominal vena cava above the renal vein

Hepatoduodenal ligament

Hepatic artery

Portal vein

Vena cava

Fig. 199

TNM Clinical Classification

T – Primary Tumour

TX   Primary tumour cannot be assessed
T0   No evidence of primary tumour
T1a   Solitary tumour less than or equal to 2 cm in greatest dimension with or without vascular invasion (Fig. 200)
T1b   Solitary tumour more than 2 cm in greatest dimension without vascular invasion
T2   Solitary tumour with vascular invasion *or* multiple tumours, none more than 5 cm in greatest dimension (Figs. 201, 202)

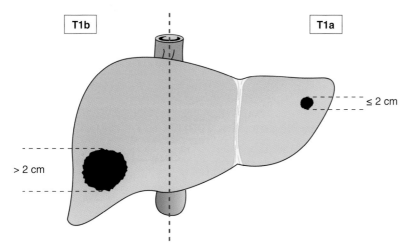

Fig. 200

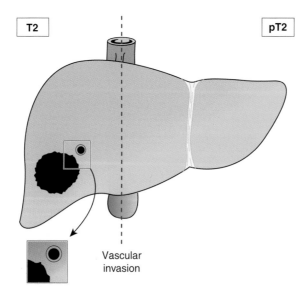

Fig. 201

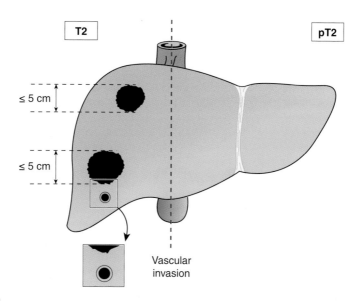

Fig. 202

T3   Multiple tumours any more than 5 cm in greatest dimension (Fig. 203)
T4   Tumour(s) involving a major branch of the portal or hepatic vein or with direct invasion of adjacent organs (including the diaphragm), other than the gallbladder, *or* with perforation of visceral peritoneum (Figs. 204, 205)

N – Regional Lymph Nodes

NX   Regional lymph nodes cannot be assessed
N0   No regional lymph node metastasis
N1   Regional lymph node metastasis (Fig. 206)

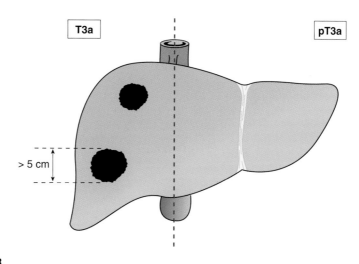

Fig. 203

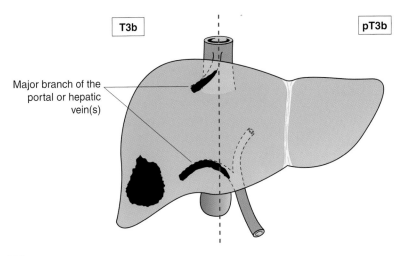

T3b   pT3b

Major branch of the
portal or hepatic
vein(s)

Fig. 204

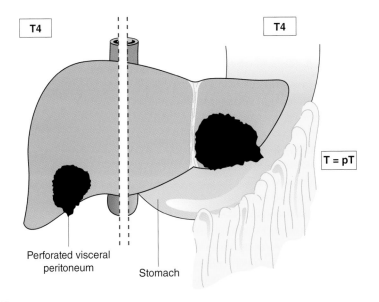

T4   T4

T = pT

Perforated visceral
peritoneum   Stomach

Fig. 205

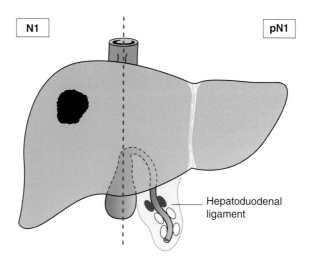

Fig. 206

M – Distant Metastasis

M0   No distant metastasis
M1   Distant metastasis

TNM Pathological Classification

The pT and pN categories correspond to the T and N categories.

pM1   Distant metastasis microscopically confirmed

Note
pM0 and pMX are not valid categories.

pN0   Histological examination of a regional lymphadenectomy specimen will ordinarily include 3 or more lymph nodes. If the lymph nodes are negative, but the number ordinarily examined is not met, classify as pN0.

Summary

Liver – Hepatocellular Carcinoma

T1a	Solitary tumour ≤ 2 cm in greatest dimension with or without vascular invasion
T1b	Solitary tumour > 2 cm in greatest dimension without vascular invasion
T2	Solitary tumour with vascular invasion > 2 cm dimension *or* multiple tumours, none > 5 cm
T3	Multiple tumours any more than 5 cm in greatest dimension
T4	Tumour(s) involving a major branch of the portal or hepatic vein or with direct invasion of adjacent organs (including the diaphragm), other than the gallbladder, *or* with perforation of visceral peritoneum

N – Regional Lymph Nodes

NX	Regional lymph nodes cannot be assessed
N0	No regional lymph node metastasis
N1	Regional lymph node metastasis

M – Distant Metastasis

M0	No distant metastasis
M1	Distant metastasis

LIVER – INTRAHEPATIC BILE DUCTS (ICD-O-3 C22.1)

Rules for Classification

The staging system applies only to intrahepatic cholangiocarcinoma, cholangiocellular carcinoma, and combined hepatocellular and cholangiocarcinoma (mixed hepatocellular/cholangiocellular carcinoma)

Regional Lymph Nodes

For right liver intrahepatic cholangiocarcinoma, the regional lymph nodes include the hilar (common bile duct, hepatic artery, portal vein and cystic duct), periduodenal and peripancreatic lymph nodes.

For left liver intrahepatic cholangiocarcinoma, regional lymph nodes include hilar and gastrohepatic lymph nodes.

For intrahepatic cholangiocarcinoma, spread to the coeliac and/or periaortic and caval lymph nodes are distant metastases (M1).

TNM Clinical Classification

T – Primary Tumour

TX   Primary tumour cannot be assessed
T0   No evidence of primary tumour
Tis   Carcinoma in situ (intraductal tumour)

      T1a   Solitary tumour 5 cm or less in greatest dimension without vascular invasion (Fig. 207)

      T1b   Solitary tumour more than 5 cm in greatest dimension without vascular invasion (Fig. 207)

      T2   Solitary tumour with intrahepatic vascular invasion or multiple tumours, with or without vascular invasion (Figs. 208, 209)

      T3   Tumour perforating the visceral peritoneum (Fig. 210)

      T4   Tumour involving local extrahepatic structures by hepatic invasion (Fig. 210)

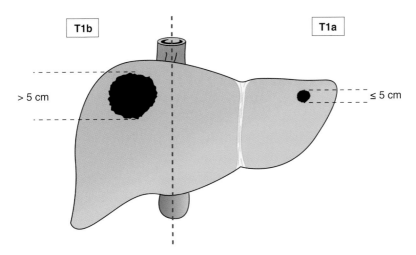

Fig. 207

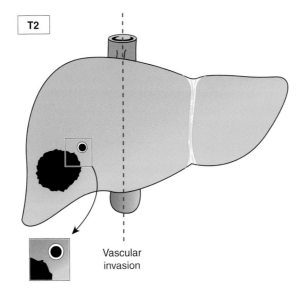

Fig. 208

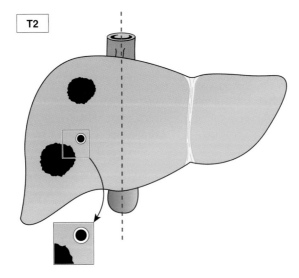

Fig. 209

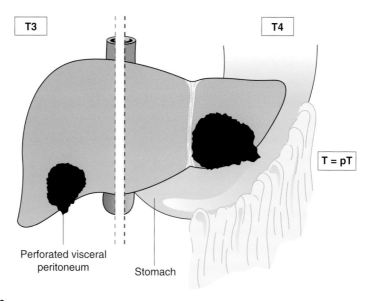

Fig. 210

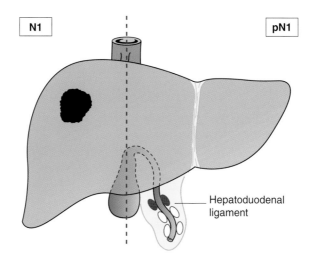

Fig. 211

N – Regional Lymph Nodes

NX   Regional lymph nodes cannot be assessed
N0   No regional lymph node metastasis
N1   Regional lymph node metastasis (Fig. 211)

M – Distant Metastasis

M0   No distant metastasis
M1   Distant metastasis

TNM Pathological Classification

The pT and pN categories correspond to the T and N categories.

pM1   Distant metastasis microscopically confirmed

Note
pM0 and pMX are not valid categories.

pN0   Histological examination of a regional lymphadenectomy specimen will ordinarily include 3 or more lymph nodes. If the regional lymph nodes are negative, but the number ordinarily examined is not met, classify as pN0.

Summary

Intrahepatic Bile Ducts	
T1a	Solitary tumour ≤ 5 cm without vascular invasion
T1b	Solitary tumour > 5 cm without vascular invasion
T2	Solitary tumour with intrahepatic vascular invasion *or* multiple tumours, with or without vascular invasion
T3	Tumour perforating the visceral peritoneum
T4	Tumour involving local extrahepatic structures by hepatic invasion
N1	Regional
M1	Distant

GALLBLADDER (ICD-O-3 C23.9 and C24.0)

Rules for Classification

The classification applies only to carcinomas of the gallbladder and cystic duct. There should be histological confirmation of the disease.

Regional Lymph Nodes (Fig. 216)

Regional lymph nodes are limited to the hepatic hilus (including nodes along the common bile duct, hepatic artery, portal vein and cystic duct).

Coeliac, periduodenal, peripancreatic and superior mesenteric artery node involvement is considered distant metastasis (M1).

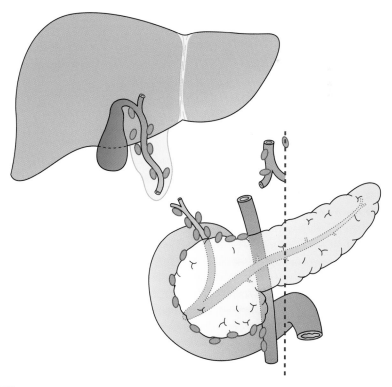

Fig. 212

TNM Clinical Classification

T – Primary Tumour

TX　　Primary tumour cannot be assessed
T0　　No evidence of primary tumour
Tis　　Carcinoma in situ
T1　　Tumour invades lamina propria or muscular layer (Fig. 213)
　　　　T1a　　Tumour invades lamina propria
　　　　T1b　　Tumour invades muscular layer
T2　　Tumour invades perimuscular connective tissue; no extension beyond serosa or into liver (Fig. 214)
　　　　T2a　　Tumour invades perimuscular connective tissue on the peritoneal side with no extension to the serosa
　　　　T2b　　Tumour invades perimuscular connective tissue on the hepatic side with no extension into the liver

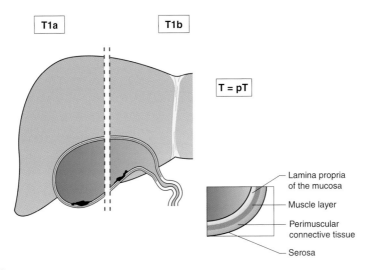

Fig. 213

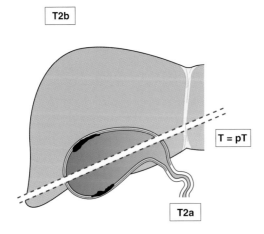

Fig. 214

T3   Tumour perforates the serosa (visceral peritoneum) and/or directly invades the liver and/or one other adjacent organ or structure, such as stomach, duodenum, colon, pancreas, omentum, extrahepatic bile ducts (Figs. 215, 216)

T4   Tumour invades main portal vein or hepatic artery or invades two or more extrahepatic organs or structures (Figs. 217, 218)

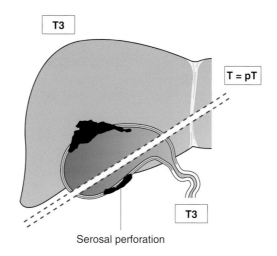

Fig. 215

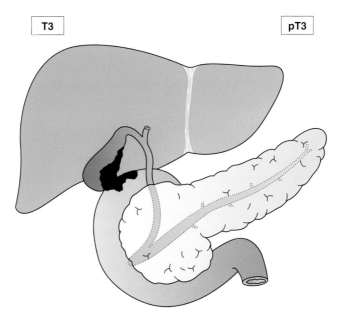

Fig. 216

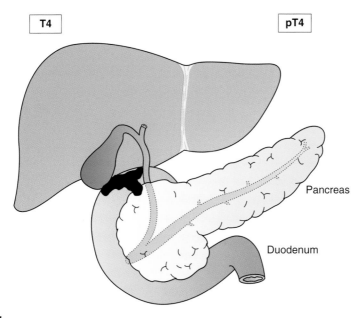

T4

pT4

Pancreas

Duodenum

Fig. 217

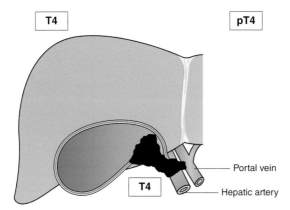

T4

pT4

T4

Portal vein

Hepatic artery

Fig. 218

N – Regional Lymph Nodes (Figs. 219, 220)

NX   Regional lymph nodes cannot be assessed
N0   No regional lymph node metastasis
N1   Metastases to 1-3 nodes
N2   Metastases to 4 or more nodes

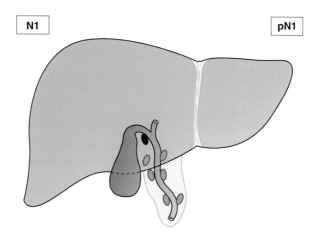

N1   pN1

Fig. 219

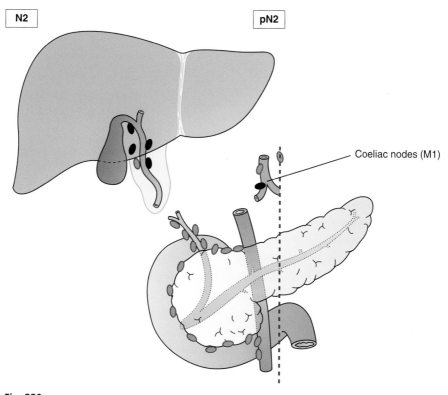

N2   pN2

Coeliac nodes (M1)

Fig. 220

M – Distant Metastasis

M0   No distant metastasis

M1   Distant metastasis

TNM Pathological Classification

The pT and pN categories correspond to the T and N categories.

pM1   Distant metastasis microscopically confirmed

Note

pM0 and pMX are not valid categories.

pN0   Histological examination of a regional lymphadenectomy specimen will ordinarily include 3 or more lymph nodes. If the regional lymph nodes are negative, but the number ordinarily examined is not met, classify as pN0.

Summary

Gallbladder		
T1	Lamina propria or muscular layer	
	T1a	Lamina propria
	T1b	Muscular layer
T2	Perimuscular connective tissue	
	T2a	On the peritoneal side with no extension to the serosa
	T2b	On the hepatic side with no extension into the liver
T3	Serosa, one organ and/or liver	
T4	Portal vein, hepatic artery or two or more extrahepatic organs	
N1	Metastases to 1-3 nodes	
N2	Metastases to 4 or more nodes	
M1	Distant (including lymph nodes defined as distant)	

EXTRAHEPATIC BILE DUCTS – PERIHILAR (ICD-O-3 C24.0)

Rules for Classification

The classification applies to carcinomas of the extrahepatic bile ducts of perihilar localization (Klatskin tumour). Included are the right, left and common hepatic ducts.

Anatomical Sites and Subsites (Fig. 221)

Perihilar cholangiocarcinomas are tumours located in the extrahepatic biliary tree proximal to the origin of the cystic duct.

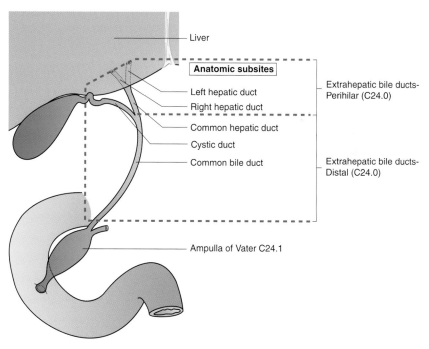

Liver

Anatomic subsites

Left hepatic duct
Right hepatic duct

Common hepatic duct

Cystic duct

Common bile duct

Extrahepatic bile ducts-Perihilar (C24.0)

Extrahepatic bile ducts-Distal (C24.0)

Ampulla of Vater C24.1

Fig. 221

Regional Lymph Nodes

The regional nodes are the hilar and pericholedochal nodes in the hepatoduodenal ligament.

TNM Clinical Classification

T – Primary Tumour

TX   Primary tumour cannot be assessed
T0   No evidence of primary tumour
Tis   Carcinoma in situ
T1   Tumour confined to the bile duct, with extension up to the muscle layer or fibrous tissue (Fig. 222)
T2a   Tumour invades beyond the wall of the bile duct to surrounding adipose tissue (Fig. 223)
T2b   Tumour invades adjacent hepatic parenchyma (Fig. 224)
T3   Tumour invades unilateral branches of the portal vein or hepatic artery (Fig. 225a)
T4   Tumour invades the main portal vein or its branches bilaterally; or the common hepatic artery; or the second-order biliary radicals bilaterally; or unilateral second-order biliary radicals with contralateral portal vein or hepatic artery involvement (Fig. 225b)

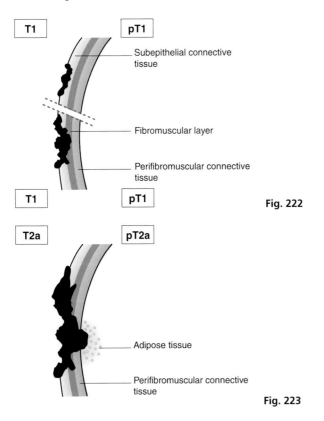

Fig. 222

Fig. 223

T2b   pT2b

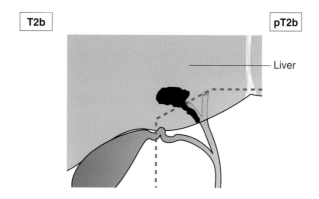

Liver

Fig. 224

(a)

T3   pT3

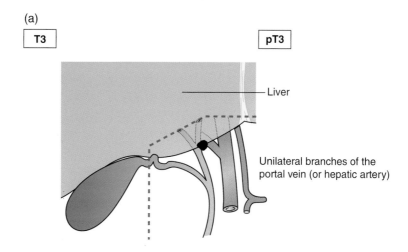

Liver

Unilateral branches of the
portal vein (or hepatic artery)

(b)

T4   pT4

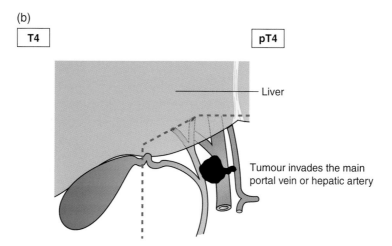

Liver

Tumour invades the main
portal vein or hepatic artery

Fig. 225

N – Regional Lymph Nodes

NX   Regional lymph nodes cannot be assessed
N0   No regional lymph node metastasis
N1   Metastases to 1 to 3 regional lymph nodes
N2   Metastases to 4 or more regional nodes

M – Distant Metastasis

M0   No distant metastasis
M1   Distant metastasis

TNM Pathological Classification

The pT and pN categories correspond to the T and N categories.

pM1   Distant metastasis microscopically confirmed

Note
pM0 and pMX are not valid categories.

pN0   Histological examination of a regional lymphadenectomy specimen will ordinarily include 15 or more lymph nodes. If the regional lymph nodes are negative, but the number ordinarily examined is not met, classify as pN0.

Summary

Perihilar Bile Ducts	
T1	Ductal wall
T2a	Beyond ductal wall
T2b	Adjacent hepatic parenchyma
T3	Unilateral branches of portal vein or hepatic artery
T4	Main portal vein; bilateral branches; common hepatic artery; second-order biliary radicals bilaterally; unilateral second-order biliary radicals with contralateral portal vein or hepatic artery involvement
	N1 Metastases to 1–3 regional lymph nodes
	N2 Metastases to 4 or more regional nodes
M1	Distant metastasis

EXTRAHEPATIC BILE DUCTS – DISTAL (ICD-O-3 C24.0)

Rules for Classification

The classification applies to carcinomas of the extrahepatic bile ducts distal to the insertion of the cystic duct. Cystic duct carcinoma is included under gallbladder.

Regional Lymph Nodes

The regional lymph nodes are along the common bile duct, hepatic artery, back towards the coeliac trunk, posterior and anterior pancreaticoduodenal nodes, and nodes along the superior mesenteric artery.

TNM Clinical Classification

T – Primary Tumour

TX	Primary tumour cannot be assessed
T0	No evidence of primary tumour
Tis	Carcinoma in situ
T1	Tumour invades bile duct wall to a depth of less than 5 mm (Fig. 226)
T2	Tumour invades bile duct wall to a depth of 5 mm up to 12 mm (Fig. 226)
T3	Tumour invades bile duct wall to a depth of more than 12 mm (Fig. 227)
T4	Tumour involves the coeliac axis or the superior mesenteric artery (Fig. 228)

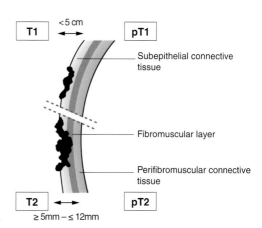

Fig. 226

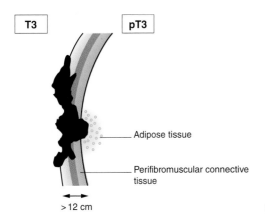

Adipose tissue

Perifibromuscular connective tissue

> 12 cm

Fig. 227

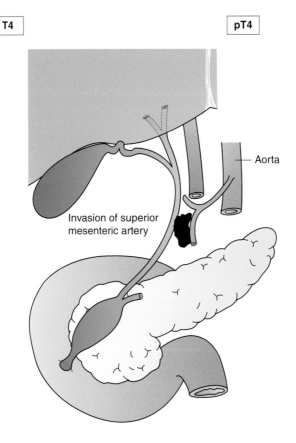

Aorta

Invasion of superior mesenteric artery

Fig. 228

N – Regional Lymph Nodes

NX   Regional lymph nodes cannot be assessed
N1   Metastases to 1 to 3 regional nodes
N2   Metastases to 4 or more regional nodes

M – Distant Metastasis

M0 No distant metastasis
M1 Distant metastasis

TNM Pathological Classification

The pT and pN categories correspond to the T and N categories.

pM1 Distant metastasis microscopically confirmed

Note
pM0 and pMX are not valid categories.

pN0 Histological examination of a regional lymphadenectomy specimen will ordinarily
include 12 or more lymph nodes. If the regional lymph nodes are negative, but
the number ordinarily examined is not met, classify as pN0.

Summary

Distal Extrahepatic Bile Ducts		
T1	Tumour invades bile duct bile duct < 5 mm	
T2	Tumour invades bile duct bile duct ≥ 5 mm to ≤ 12 mm	
T3	Tumour invades bile duct bile duct wall to > 12 mm	
T4	Coeliac axis or superior mesenteric artery	
N1	N1	Metastases to 1–3 regional nodes
	N2	Metastases to 4 or more regional nodes
M1	Distant	

AMPULLA OF VATER (ICD-O-3 C24.1) (FIG. 229)

Rules for Classification

The classification applies only to carcinomas. There should be histological confirmation of the disease.

Regional Lymph Nodes (Fig. 230)

The regional lymph nodes are the same as for the head of the pancreas and are the lymph nodes along the anterior and posterior pancreaticoduodenal vessels the superior mesenteric vein and right lateral wall of the superior mesenteric artery, proximal mesenteric vessels, the common hepatic artery, coeliac axis, pyloric, infrapyloric, subpyloric vessels, portal vein and common bile duct (not shown).

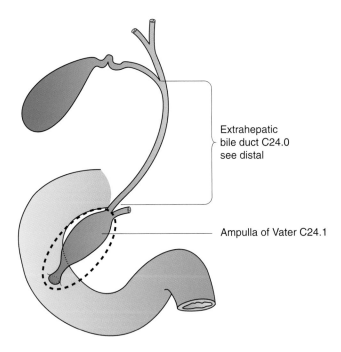

Extrahepatic bile duct C24.0 see distal

Ampulla of Vater C24.1

Fig. 229

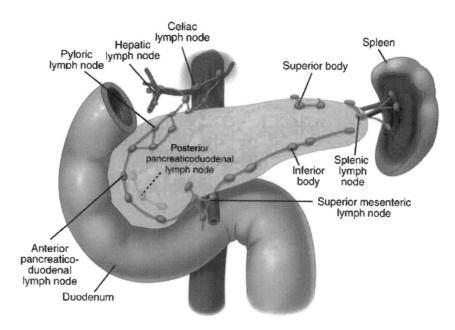

Fig. 230 Source: From F. Charles Brunicardi et al. (2015) *Schwartz's Principles of Surgery,* 10th edition, McGraw Hill Education. © 2015 McGraw Hill Education.

Note

The splenic lymph nodes and those of the tail of the pancreas are *not* regional; metastases to these lymph nodes are coded M1.

TNM Clinical Classification

T – Primary Tumour

TX	Primary tumour cannot be assessed
T0	No evidence of primary tumour
Tis	Carcinoma in situ
T1a	Tumour limited to ampulla of Vater or sphincter of Oddi (Fig. 231)
T1b	Tumour invades beyond the sphincter of Oddi (perisphincteric invasion) and/or into the duodenal submucosa (Fig. 232)
T2	Tumour invades the muscularis propria of the duodenum

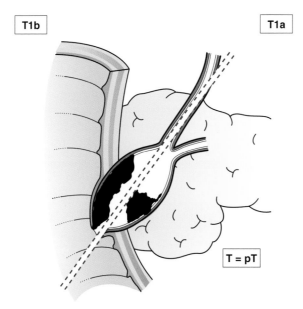

Fig. 231

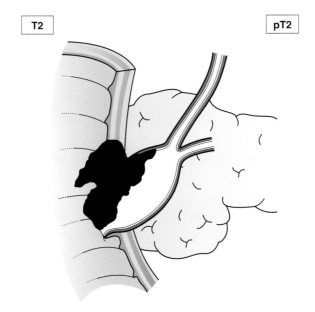

Fig. 232

T3   Tumour invades pancreas or peripancreatic tissue (Fig. 233)
    T3a   Tumour invades no more than 0.5 cm into the pancreas
    T3b   Tumour invades more than 0.5 cm into the pancreas or extends into
           peripancreatic tissue or duodenal serosa, but without involvement of the
           coeliac axis or the superior mesenteric artery
T4   Tumour with vascular involvement of the superior mesenteric artery or coeliac
    axis, or portal venous involvement that cannot be reconstructed (Fig. 234)

T3

pT3

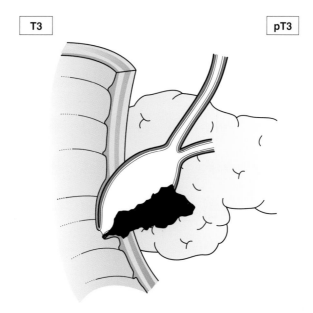

Fig. 233

T4

pT4

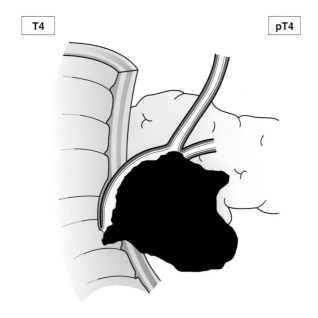

Fig. 234

N – Regional Lymph Nodes

NX   Regional lymph nodes cannot be assessed
N0   No regional lymph node metastasis
N1   Metastasis in 1 or 3 regional lymph nodes (Fig. 235)
N2   Metastasis in 4 or more regional lymph nodes (Fig. 236)

M – Distant Metastasis

M0   No distant metastasis
M1   Distant metastasis (Fig. 237)

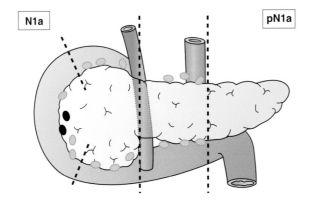

Fig. 235

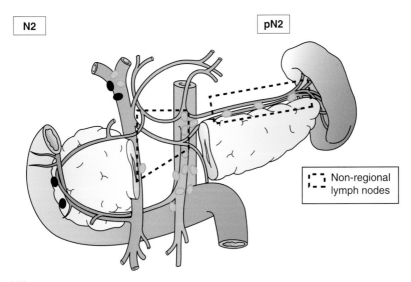

Fig. 236

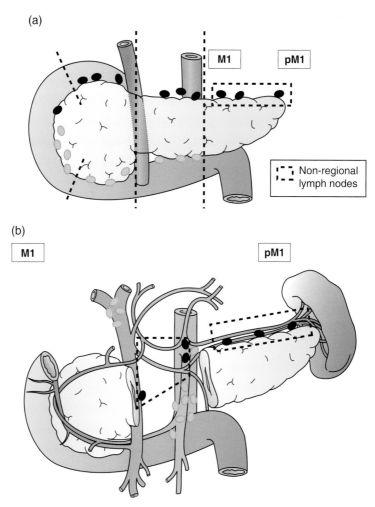

(a)

M1   pM1

Non-regional
lymph nodes

(b)

M1   pM1

Fig. 237

TNM Pathological Classification

The pT and pN categories correspond to the T and N categories.

pM1   Distant metastasis microscopically confirmed

Note
pM0 and pMX are not valid categories.

pN0   Histological examination of a regional lymphadenectomy specimen will ordinarily
include 10 or more lymph nodes. If the lymph nodes are negative, but the
number ordinarily examined is not met, classify as pN0.

Summary

Ampulla of Vater	
N1	Regional
M1	Distant
T1a	Tumour limited to ampulla or sphincter
T1b	Tumour invades beyond ampulla or sphincter and/or into the duodenal submucosa
T2	Tumour invades the muscularis propria
T3a	Tumour invades ≤ 0.5 cm into the pancreas
T3b	Tumour invades > 0.5 cm into the pancreas or extends into peripancreatic tissue or duodenal serosa
T4	Tumour with vascular involvement
N1	Metastasis in 1 to 3 regional nodes
N2	Metastasis in ≥4
M1	Distant

PANCREAS (ICD-O-3 C25)

Rules for Classification

The classification applies to carcinomas of the exocrine pancreas and pancreatic neuroendocrine tumours, including carcinoids. There should be histological or cytological confirmation of the disease.

Anatomical Subsites (Fig. 238)

C25.0	Head of pancreas
C25.1	Body of pancreas
C25.2	Tail of pancreas
C25.3	Pancreatic duct
C25.4	Islets of Langerhans (endocrine pancreas)

Notes

[1]Tumours of the head of the pancreas are those arising to the right of the left border of the superior mesenteric vein. The uncinate process is considered as part of the head.

[2]Tumours of the body are those arising between the left border of the superior mesenteric vein and the left border of the aorta.

[3]Tumours of the tail are those arising between the left border of the aorta and the hilum of the spleen.

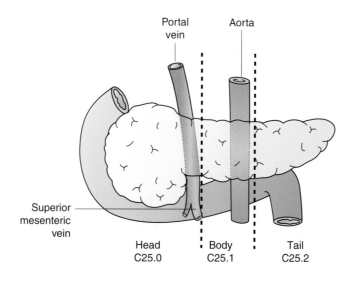

Fig. 238

Regional Lymph Nodes (Fig. 239)

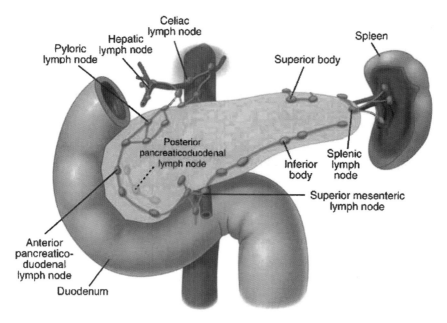

Fig. 239   Source: From F. Charles Brunicardi et al., *Schwartz's Principles of Surgery*, 10th edition, 2015, McGraw Hill Education. © 2015 McGraw Hill Education

The regional lymph nodes for tumours in the head and neck of the pancreas are the lymph nodes along the anterior and posterior pancreaticoduodenal vessels, the superior mesenteric vein and right lateral wall of the superior mesenteric artery, proximal mesenteric vessels, the common hepatic artery, coeliac axis, pyloric, infrapyloric, subpyloric vessels, portal vein and common bile duct (not shown).

The regional lymph nodes for tumours in body and tail are the lymph nodes along the common hepatic artery, coeliac axis, splenic artery and splenic hilum, as well as retroperitoneal nodes and lateral aortic nodes.

TNM Clinical Classification

T – Primary Tumour

TX   Primary tumour cannot be assessed
T0   No evidence of primary tumour
Tis   Carcinoma in situ*
T1   Tumour 2 cm or less in greatest dimension (Fig. 240)
      T1a   Tumour 0.5 cm or less in greatest dimension
      T1b   Tumour greater than 0.5 cm and no more than 1 cm in greatest dimension
      T1c   Tumour greater than 1 cm but no more than 2 cm in greatest dimension

T2   Tumour limited to pancreas, more than 2 cm but no more than 4 cm in greatest dimension (Fig. 240)

T3   Tumour limited to pancreas, more than 4 cm in greatest dimension (Fig. 241)

T4   Tumour involves coeliac axis, superior mesenteric artery and/or common hepatic artery (Fig. 242)

Note

*Tis also includes the "PanIN-III" classification.

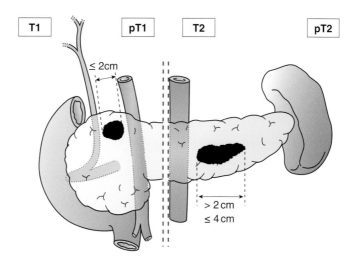

Fig. 240

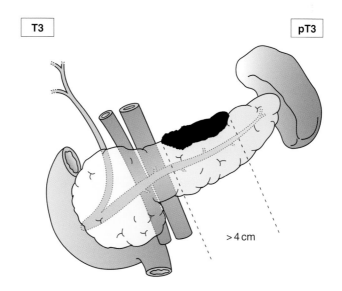

Fig. 241

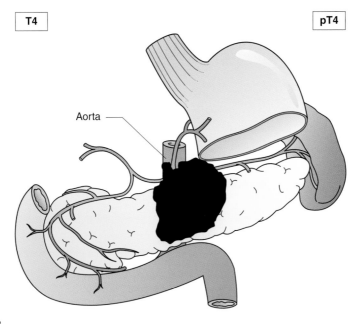

Fig. 242

N – Regional Lymph Nodes

NX   Regional lymph nodes cannot be assessed
N0   No regional lymph node metastasis
N0   No regional lymph node metastasis
N1   Metastases in 1 to 3 regional lymph node(s) (Fig. 243)
N2   Metastases in 4 or more regional lymph nodes (Fig. 244)

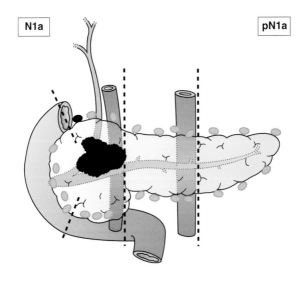

Fig. 243

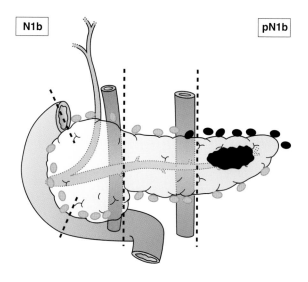

N1b   pN1b

Fig. 244

M – Distant Metastasis

M0   No distant metastasis
M1   Distant metastasis

TNM Pathological Classification

The pT and pN categories correspond to the T and N categories.

pM1   Distant metastasis microscopically confirmed

Note
pM0 and pMX are not valid categories.

pN0   Histological examination of a regional lymphadenectomy specimen will ordinarily
include 12 or more lymph nodes. If the lymph nodes are negative, but the
number ordinarily examined is not met, classify as pN0.

Summary

Pancreas	
T1a	Tumour $\leq$ 0.5 cm
T1b	Tumour > 0.5 cm and $\leq$ 1 cm
T1c	Tumour > 1 cm and $\leq$ 2 cm
T2	Tumour > 2 cm and $\leq$ 4 cm
T3	Tumour > 4 cm
T4	Tumour involves coeliac axis, superior mesenteric artery and/or common hepatic artery
Regional	
N1	1 to 3 nodes
N2	$\geq$ 4 nodes
M1	Distant

WELL-DIFFERENTIATED NEUROENDOCRINE TUMOURS OF THE GASTROINTESTINAL TRACT

Rules for Classification

This classification system applies to well-differentiated neuroendocrine tumours (carcinoid tumours and atypical carcinoid tumours) of the gastrointestinal tract, including the pancreas. Neuroendocrine tumours of the lung should be classified according to criteria for carcinoma of the lung. Merkel cell carcinoma of the skin has a separate classification.

High-grade neuroendocrine carcinomas are excluded and should be classified according to criteria for classifying carcinomas at the respective site.

Histopathological Grading

The following grading scheme has been proposed for all gastrointestinal neuroendocrine tumours (carcinoids):

Grade	Mitotic count (per 10 HPF)[1]	Ki-67 index (%)[2]
G1	< 2	≤ 2
G2	2–20	3–20
G3	> 20	> 20

Notes
[1] 10 HPF: high power field = 2 mm², at least 40 fields (at 40× magnification) evaluated in areas of highest mitotic density.
[2] MIB1 antibody; % of 500–2,000 tumour cells in areas of highest nuclear labelling.
All Grade 3/high-grade tumours should be classified according to criteria for classifying carcinoma at the respective sites.

Stomach

TNM Clinical Classification

T – Primary Tumour

TX   Primary tumour cannot be assessed
T0   No evidence of primary tumour
T1   Tumour invades the mucosa or submucosa and is no greater than 1 cm in greatest dimension (Fig. 245)

T2   Tumour invades muscularis propria or is more than 1 cm in greatest dimension
        (Fig. 245)

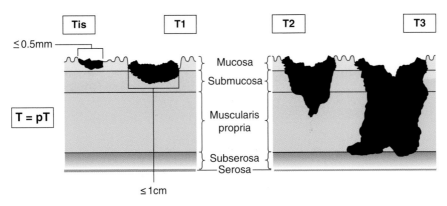

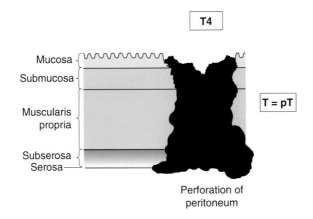

Fig. 245

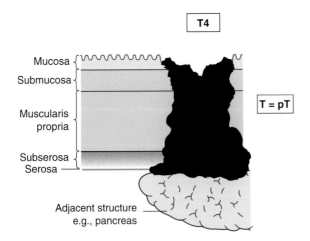

Fig. 246

Fig. 247

T3   Tumour invades subserosa (Fig. 245)

T4   Tumour perforates visceral peritoneum (serosa) (Fig. 246) or other organs or adjacent structures (Fig. 247)

Note

For any T, add (m) for multiple tumours.

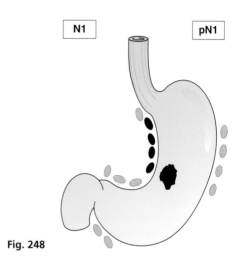

Fig. 248

N – Regional Lymph Nodes

NX   Regional lymph nodes cannot be assessed

N0   No regional lymph node metastasis

N1   Regional lymph node metastasis (Fig. 248)

M – Distant Metastasis

M0   No distant metastasis

M1   Distant metastasis

    M1a   Hepatic metastasis(es) only

    M1b   Extrahepatic metastasis(es) only

    M1c   Hepatic and extrahepatic metastases

Duodenum, Ampulla, Jejunum, Ileum

TNM Clinical Classification

T – Primary Tumour

TX   Primary tumour cannot be assessed
T0   No evidence of primary tumour
T1   *Ampullary*: Tumour 1 cm or less in greatest dimension and confined within the sphincter of Oddi
      Duodenal, Jejunum and Ileum: Tumour invades mucosa or submucosa and 1 cm or less in greatest dimension (Fig. 249)
T2   *Ampullary*: Tumour invades through sphincter into duodenal submucosa or muscularis propria, or more than 1 cm in greatest dimension (Fig. 249)
      Duodenal, Jejunum and Ileum: Tumour invades muscularis propria or is more than 1 cm in greatest dimension (Fig. 249)
      Jejunum or Ileum: Tumour invades through the muscularis propria into subseral tissue, without penetration of the overlying serosa (Fig. 250)
T3   *Ampullary, Duodenum*: Tumour invades pancreas or peripacreatic adipose tissue (Fig. 251)
T4   Tumour perforates visceral peritoneum (serosa) or invades other organs or adjacent structures (Fig. 252)

Note
Tumour limited to ampulla of Vater for ampullary gangliocytic paraganglioma.
For any T, add (m) for multiple tumours.

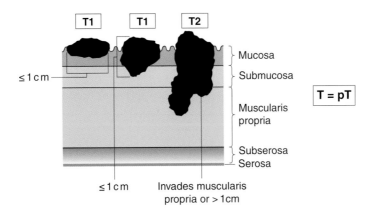

Fig. 249

T3

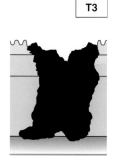

Fig. 250

T3

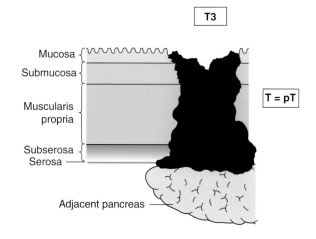

T = pT

Fig. 251

T4

pT4

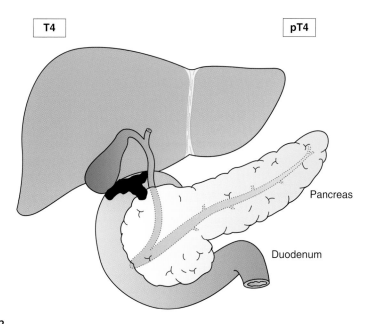

Fig. 252

N – Regional Lymph Nodes: Ampullary and Duodenum

NX   Regional lymph nodes cannot be assessed
N0   No regional lymph node metastasis
N1   Regional lymph node metastasis

N – Regional Lymph Nodes: Jejunum/Ileum

NX   Regional lymph nodes cannot be assessed
N0   No regional lymph node metastasis
N1   Less than 12 regional nodes without mesenteric mass(es) greater than 2 cm in greatest dimension
N2   More than 12 regional nodes and/or mesenteric mass(es) greater than 2 cm in greatest dimension

M – Distant Metastasis

M0   No distant metastasis
M1   Distant metastasis
      M1a   Hepatic metastasis(es) only
      M1b   Extrahepatic metastasis(es) only
      M1c   Hepatic and extrahepatic metastases

Appendix

TNM Clinical Classification

T – Primary Tumour[1]

TX   Primary tumour cannot be assessed
T0   No evidence of primary tumour
T1   Tumour 2 cm or less in greatest dimension (Fig. 253)
T2   Tumour more than 2 cm but not more than 4 cm in greatest dimension (Fig. 254)
T3   Tumour more than 4 cm or with subserosal invasion or with involvement of the mesoappendix (Fig. 255)
T4   Tumour perforates peritoneum or invades other adjacent organs or structures, e.g., abdominal wall and skeletal muscle[2] (Figs. 256, 257)

Notes
[1]Goblet cell carcinoid is classified according to the carcinoma scheme.
[2]Tumour that is adherent to other organs or structures, macroscopically, is T4. However, if no tumour is present in the adhesion, microscopically, the classification should be pT1–3 as appropriate.

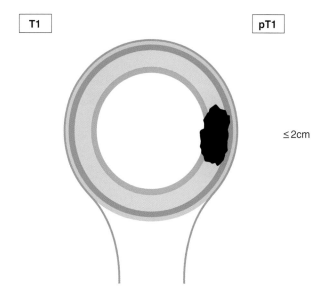

Fig. 253

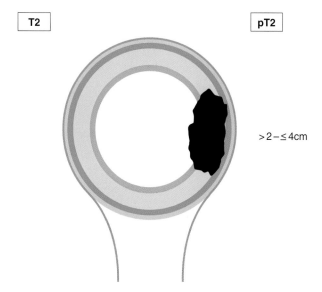

Fig. 254

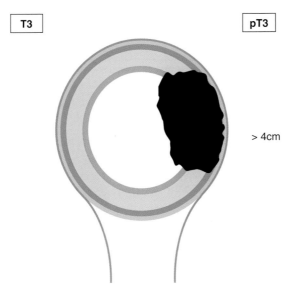

Fig. 255

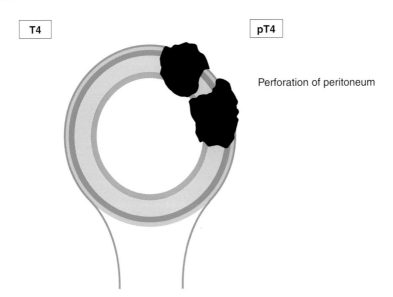

Fig. 256

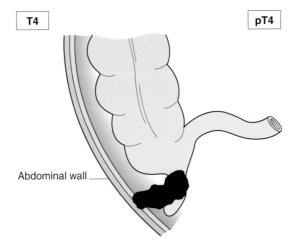

Fig. 257

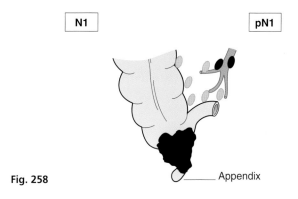

Fig. 258

N – Regional Lymph Nodes

NX   Regional lymph nodes cannot be assessed
N0   No regional lymph node metastasis
N1   Regional lymph node metastasis (Fig. 258)

M – Distant Metastasis

M0   No distant metastasis
M1   Distant metastasis
      M1a   Hepatic metastasis(es) only
      M1b   Extrahepatic metastasis(es) only
      M1c   Hepatic and extrahepatic metastases

pTNM Pathological Classification

The pT and pN categories correspond to the T and N categories.

pM1   Distant metastasis microscopically confirmed

Note
pM0 and pMX are not valid categories.

pN0   Histological examination of a regional lymphadenectomy specimen will ordinarily include 12 or more lymph nodes. If the lymph nodes are negative, but the number ordinarily examined is not met, classify as pN0.

Colon and Rectum

TNM Clinical Classification

T – Primary Tumour

TX   Primary tumour cannot be assessed
T0   No evidence of primary tumour
T1   Tumour invades lamina propria or submucosa or is no greater than 2 cm in size (Fig. 259)
T1a   Tumour less than 1 cm in size
T1b   Tumour 1 to 2 cm in size
T2   Tumour invades muscularis propria or is greater than 2 cm in size (Fig. 259)
T3   Tumour invades subserosa, or non-peritonealized pericolic or perirectal tissues (Fig. 260)
T4   Tumour perforates peritoneum or invades other organs (Fig. 261)

Note
For any T, add (m) for multiple tumours.

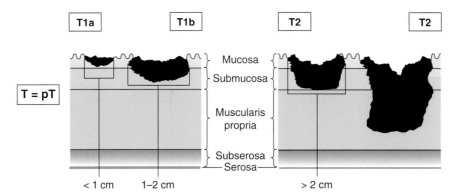

Fig. 259

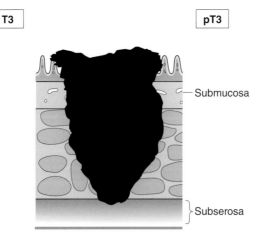

Fig. 260

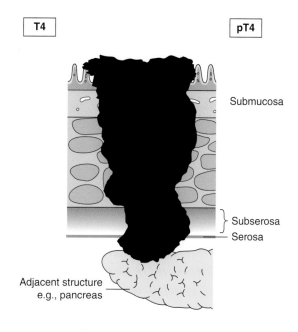

Fig. 261

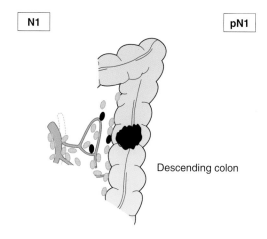

Fig. 262

N – Regional Lymph Nodes

NX   Regional lymph nodes cannot be assessed
N0   No regional lymph node metastasis
N1   Regional lymph node metastasis (Fig. 262)

M – Distant Metastasis

M0   No distant metastasis
M1   Distant metastasis
    M1a   Hepatic metastasis only
    M1b   Extrahepatic metastasis only
    M1c   Hepatic and extrahepatic metastases

Note

pM0 and pMX are not valid categories.

WELL-DIFFERENTIATED NEUROENDOCRINE TUMOURS OF THE PANCREAS

Rules for Classification

This classification system applies to well-differentiated neuroendocrine tumours (carcinoid tumours and atypical carcinoid tumours) of the pancreas.

High-grade neuroendocrine carcinomas are excluded and should be classified according to criteria for classifying carcinomas of the pancreas.

Regional lymph nodes

The regional lymph nodes correspond to those listed under the appropriate sites for carcinoma.

TNM Clinical Classification – Pancreas

T – Primary Tumour

TX   Primary tumour cannot be assessed
T0   No evidence of primary tumour
T1   Tumour limited to pancreas*, 2 cm or less in greatest dimension (Fig. 263)
T2   Tumour limited to pancreas*, more than 2 cm but less than 4 cm in greatest dimension (Fig. 263)
T3   Tumour limited to pancreas*, more than 4 cm in greatest dimension (Fig. 264) or Tumour invading duodenum or bile duct.
T4   Tumour perforates visceral peritoneum (serosa) or other organs or walls of larger vessels (Fig. 265)

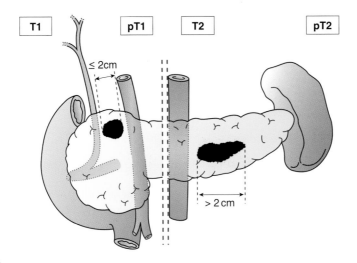

Fig. 263

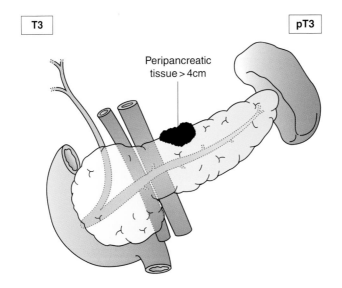

Fig. 264

T4 pT4

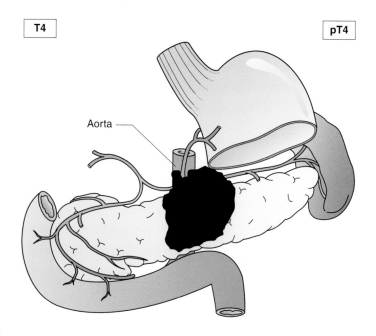

Aorta

Fig. 265

Notes

For any T, add (m) for multiple tumours.

*This includes invasion of the peripancreatic adipose tissue.

N – Regional Lymph Nodes

NX   Regional lymph nodes cannot be assessed
N0   No regional lymph node metastasis
N1   Regional lymph node metastasis

M – Distant Metastasis

M0   No distant metastasis
M1   Distant metastasis
      M1a   Hepatic metastasis(es) only
      M1b   Extrahepatic metastasis(es) only
      M1c   Hepatic and extrahepatic metastases

Summary

Stomach

T1	Mucosa or submucosa ≤ 1 cm
T2	Muscularis propria or > 1 cm
T3	Subserosa
T4	Perforates serosa; adjacent structures

Small Intestine

T1	Lamina propria or submucosa and ≤ 1 cm
T2	Muscularis propria or > 1 cm
T3	Jejunal, ileal: subserosa
	Ampullary, duodenal: invades pancreas or retroperitoneum
T4	Perforates serosa; adjacent structures

Appendix

T1	≤ 2 cm
T2	> 2–4 cm
T3	> 4 cm; invasion of mesoappendix
T4	Perforates peritoneum; other organs or structures

Colon and rectum

T1	Lamina propria or submucosa or < 2 cm
T1a	< 1 cm
T1b	1 to 2 cm
T2	Muscularis propria or > 2 cm
T3	Subserosa or pericolorectal tissue
T4	Perforates visceral peritoneum; adjacent structures

Pancreas

T1	≤ 2 cm
T2	> 2–4 cm
T3	> 4 cm
T4	Perforates peritoneum; other organs or large vessels

LUNG, PLEURAL AND THYMIC TUMOURS

The classifications apply to carcinomas of the lung, including non-small cell and small cell carcinomas, bronchopulmonary carcinoid tumours, malignant mesothelioma of pleura and thymic tumours.

Regional Lymph Nodes

The regional lymph nodes extend from the supraclavicular region to the diaphragm. Direct extension of the primary tumour into lymph nodes is classified as lymph node metastasis.

The lymph node mapping is performed according to the modified Naruke Schema (see plate 2.3 in the *TNM Supplement*, 4th edition, 2012. John Wiley & Sons).

TNM Atlas: Illustrated Guide to the TNM Classification of Malignant Tumours, Seventh Edition. Edited by James D. Brierley, Hisao Asamura, Elisabeth Van Eycken, and Brian Rous. © 2021 by UICC. Published 2021 by John Wiley & Sons Ltd.

LUNG (ICD-O C34)

Rules for Classification

The classification applies to carcinomas of the lung, including non-small cell carcinomas, small cell carcinomas and bronchopulmonary carcinoid tumours. It does not apply to sarcomas and other rare tumours.

There should be histological confirmation of the disease and division of cases by histological type.

Anatomical Subsites

1. Main bronchus (C34.0)
2. Upper lobe (C34.1)
3. Middle lobe (C34.2)
4. Lower lobe (C34.3)

Regional Lymph Nodes

The regional lymph nodes are the intrathoracic nodes (mediastinal, hilar, lobar, interlobar, segmental and subsegmental), scalene and supraclavicular lymph nodes.

TNM Clinical Classification

T – Primary Tumour

TX	Primary tumour cannot be assessed, *or* tumour proven by the presence of malignant cells in sputum or bronchial washings, but not visualized by imaging or bronchoscopy
T0	No evidence of primary tumour
Tis (AIS)	Adenocarcinoma in situ (Fig. 266)
Tis (SCC)	Squamous cell carcinoma in situ
T1	Tumour 3 cm or less in greatest dimension, surrounded by lung or visceral pleura, without bronchoscopic evidence of invasion more proximal than the lobar bronchus (i.e., not in the main bronchus)[1]

      T1mi   Minimally invasive adenocarcinoma (Fig. 266)

      T1a   Tumour 1 cm or less in greatest dimension (Fig. 266)

      T1b   Tumour more than 1 cm but not more than 2 cm in greatest dimension (Fig. 267)

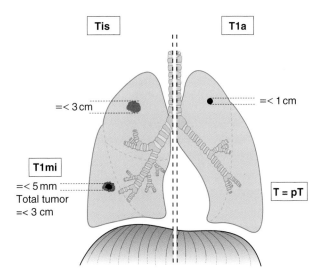

Fig. 266

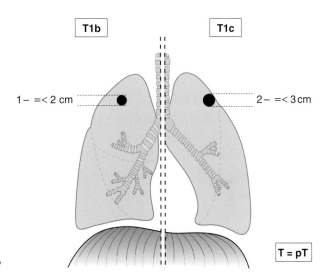

Fig. 267

T1c   Tumour more than 2 cm but not more than 3 cm in greatest dimension (Fig. 267)

T2   Tumour more than 3 cm but not more than 5 cm; or tumour with any of the following features:[2]
  - Involves main bronchus regardless of distance to the carina, but without involving the carina
  - Invades visceral pleura (Fig. 268)
  - Associated with atelectasis or obstructive pneumonitis that extends to the hilar region, either involving part of the lung or the entire lung

T2a   Tumour more than 3 cm but not more than 4 cm in greatest dimension (Fig. 269)

T2b   Tumour more than 4 cm but not more than 5 cm in greatest dimension (Fig. 269)

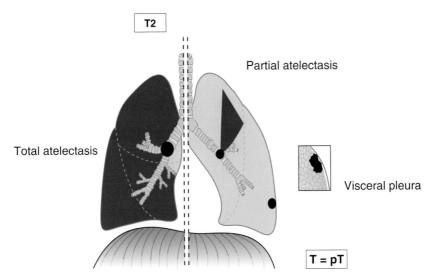

Fig. 268

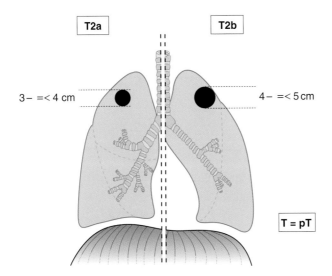

Fig. 269

T3   Tumour more than 5 cm but not more than 7 cm in greatest dimension or one
        that directly invades any of the following: chest wall (including superior sulcus
        tumours), phrenic nerve, parietal pericardium; or associated separate tumour
        nodule(s) in the same lobe as the primary (Fig. 270)

T4   Tumours more than 7 cm (Fig. 271) or one that invades any of the following:
        diaphragm (Fig. 272), mediastinum, heart (Figs. 272, 273), great vessels
        (Figs. 272, 274, 275), trachea, recurrent laryngeal nerve, oesophagus
        (Fig. 276), vertebral body (Fig. 277), carina; separate tumour nodule(s) in a
        different ipsilateral lobe to that of the primary (Fig. 271)

In tumour masses, grey colour means part-solid/non-invasive tumour; black colour
means solid/invasive tumour.

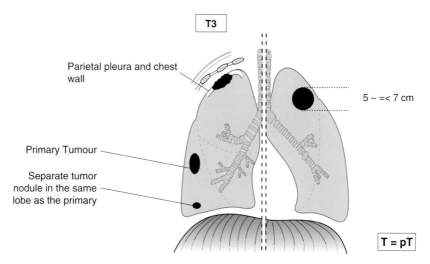

Fig. 270

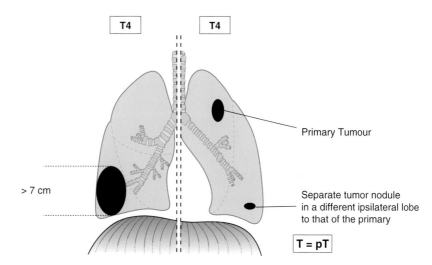

Fig. 271

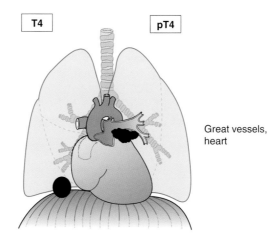

Fig. 272

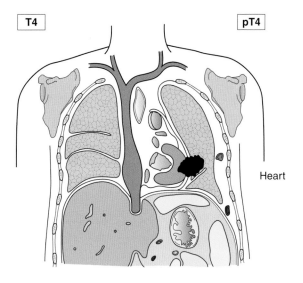

T4   pT4

Heart

Fig. 273

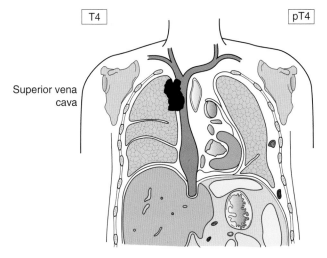

T4   pT4

Superior vena cava

Fig. 274

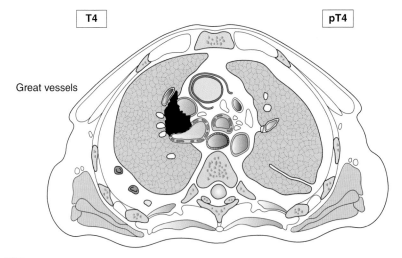

T4   pT4

Great vessels

Fig. 275

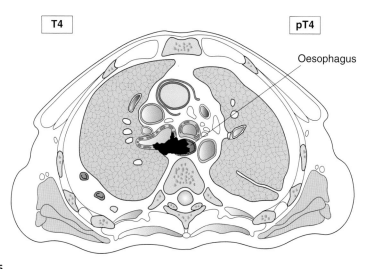

Fig. 276

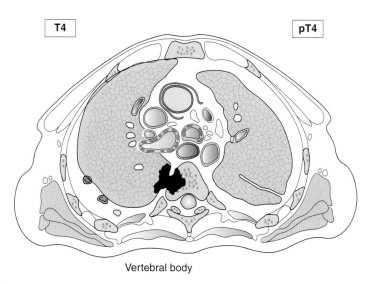

Fig. 277

N – Regional Lymph Nodes

NX   Regional lymph nodes cannot be assessed
N0   No regional lymph node metastasis
N1   Metastasis in ipsilateral peribronchial, ipsilateral interlobar and/or ipsilateral hilar lymph nodes and Intrapulmonary nodes, including involvement by direct extension (Figs. 278, 279)
N2   Metastasis in ipsilateral mediastinal and/or subcarinal lymph node(s) (Fig. 280)
N3   Metastasis in contralateral mediastinal, contralateral hilar, ipsilateral or contralateral scalene, or supraclavicular lymph node(s) (Fig. 281)

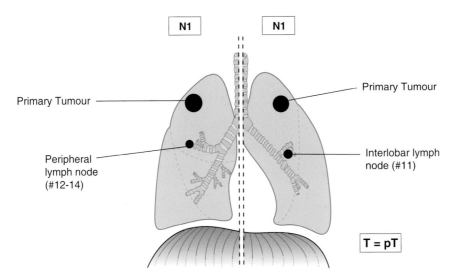

Fig. 278

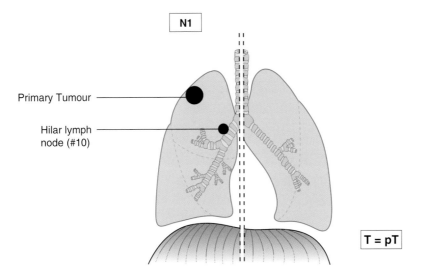

Fig. 279

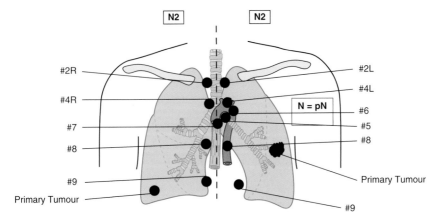

Fig. 280

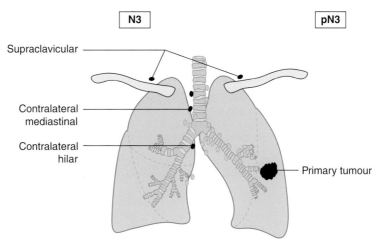

Fig. 281

M – Distant Metastasis

M0   No distant metastasis
M1   Distant metastasis

    M1a   Separate tumour nodule(s) in a contralateral lobe (Fig. 282); tumour with pleural or pericardial nodules or malignant pleural (Fig. 283) or pericardial effusion (Fig. 284)[3]

    M1b   Single extrathoracic metastasis in a single organ (Figs. 285, 286)

    M1c   Multiple extrathoracic metastases in a single or multiple organ(s) (Fig. 287)

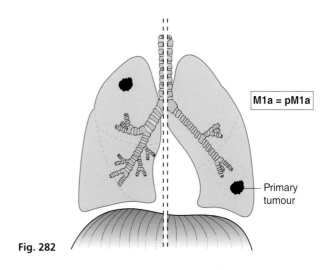

Fig. 282

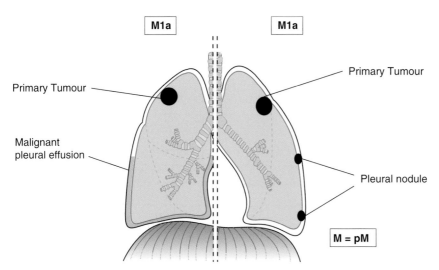

M1a   M1a

Primary Tumour

Primary Tumour

Malignant
pleural effusion

Pleural nodule

M = pM

Fig. 283

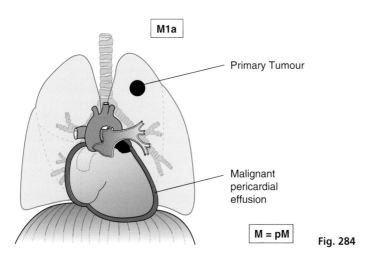

M1a

Primary Tumour

Malignant
pericardial
effusion

M = pM

Fig. 284

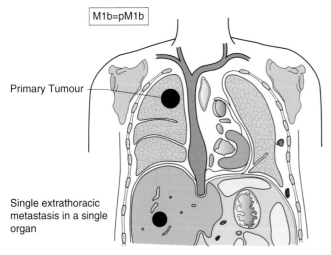

M1b=pM1b

Primary Tumour

Single extrathoracic
metastasis in a single
organ

Fig. 285

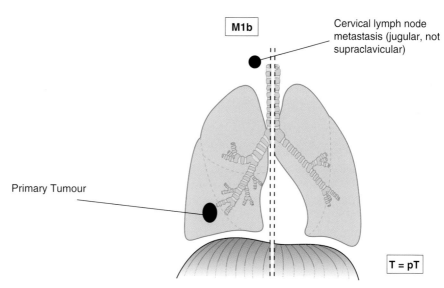

Fig. 286

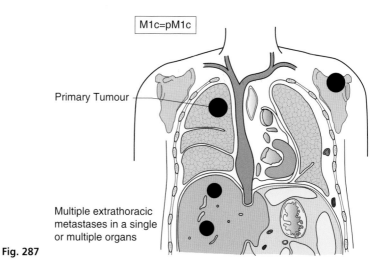

Fig. 287

Notes

[1] The uncommon superficial spreading tumour of any size with its invasive component limited to the bronchial wall, which may extend proximal to the main bronchus, is also classified as T1a.

[2] T2 tumours with these features are classified T2a if 4 cm or less, or if size cannot be determined, and T2b if greater than 4 cm but not larger than 5 cm.

[3] Most pleural (pericardial) effusions with lung cancer are due to tumour. In a few patients, however, multiple microscopical examinations of pleural (pericardial) fluid are negative for tumour, and the fluid is non-bloody and is not an exudate. Where these elements and clinical judgement dictate that the effusion is not related to the tumour, the effusion should be excluded as a staging element.

pTNM Pathological Classification

The pT and pN categories correspond to the T and N categories.

pM1   Distant metastasis microscopically confirmed

Note
pM0 and pMX are not valid categories.

pN0   Histological examination of hilar and mediastinal lymphadenectomy specimen(s) will ordinarily include 6 or more lymph nodes/stations. Three of these nodes/stations should be mediastinal, including the subcarinal nodes, and three from N1 nodes/stations. Labelling according to the IASLC chart and table of definitions given in the *TNM Supplement* is desirable. If all the lymph nodes examined are negative, but the number ordinarily examined is not met, classify as pN0.

Summary

Lung		
TX	Positive cytology only	
Tis (AIS), Tis (SCC)		
T1	≤ 3 cm	
	T1mi	
	T1a	≤ 1 cm
	T1b	> 1–2 cm
	T1c	> 2–3 cm
T2	Main bronchus, invades visceral pleura, partial or total atelectasis	
	T2a	> 3–4 cm
	T2b	> 4–5 cm
T3	> 5–7 cm; parietal pleura, chest wall, pericardium, phrenic nerve, separate nodule(s) in same lobe	
T4	Diaphragm, mediastinum, heart, great vessels, carina, trachea, oesophagus, vertebral body; separate tumour nodule(s) in a different ipsilateral lobe	
N1	Ipsilateral peribronchial, ipsilateral interlobar, ipsilateral hilar	
N2	Ipsilateral mediastinal subcarinal	
N3	Contralateral mediastinal or hilar, scalene or supraclavicular	
M1	Distant metastasis	
	M1a	Separate tumour nodule(s) in a contralateral lung; pleural or pericardial nodules or malignant pleural or pericardial effusion
	M1b	Single extrathoracic metastasis in a single organ
	M1c	Multiple extrathoracic metastases in a single or multiple organ(s)

PLEURAL MESOTHELIOMA (ICD-O-3 C38.4)

Rules for Classification

The classification applies only to malignant mesothelioma of the pleura. There should be histological confirmation of the disease.

Regional Lymph Nodes

The regional lymph nodes are the intrathoracic, internal mammary, scalene and supraclavicular nodes.

TNM Clinical Classification

T – Primary Tumour

TX   Primary tumour cannot be assessed

T0   No evidence of primary tumour

T1   Tumour involves ipsilateral parietal pleura only, with or without involvement of visceral, mediastinal or diaphragmatic pleura (Figs. 288, 289, 290a)

T2   Tumour involves the ipsilateral pleura (parietal or visceral pleura), with at least one of the following:
- Invasion of diaphragmatic muscle (Fig. 290b)
- Invasion of lung parenchyma (Fig. 290b)

T3   Tumour involves ipsilateral pleura (parietal or visceral pleura), with at least one of the following:
- Invasion of endothoracic fascia (Fig. 291a)
- Solitary focus of tumour invading soft tissues of the chest wall (Fig. 291b)
- Invasion into mediastinal fat (Fig. 292a)
- Non-transmural involvement of the pericardium (Fig. 292b)

T4   Tumour involves ipsilateral pleura (parietal or visceral pleura), with at least one of the following:
- Chest wall, with or without associated rib destruction (diffuse or multifocal) (Fig. 293)
- Peritoneum (via direct transdiaphragmatic extension) (Figs. 294, 295a)
- Contralateral pleura (Fig. 296)
- Mediastinal organs (oesophagus, trachea, heart, great vessels) (Figs. 295b, 296)
- Vertebra, neuroforamen, spinal cord (Fig. 296)
- Internal surface of the pericardium (transmural invasion with or without a pericardial effusion) or involvement of the myometrium (Fig. 295b, 296)

193

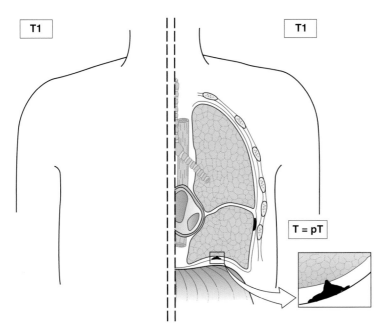

Fig. 288

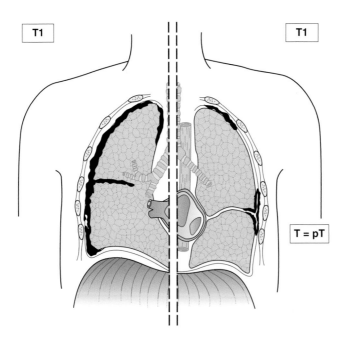

Fig. 289

Lung, pleural, thymic

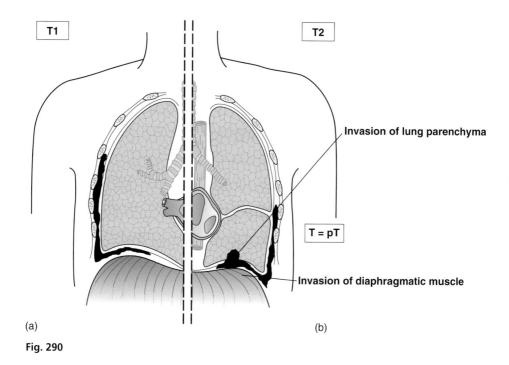

T1

T2

Invasion of lung parenchyma

T = pT

Invasion of diaphragmatic muscle

(a)

(b)

Fig. 290

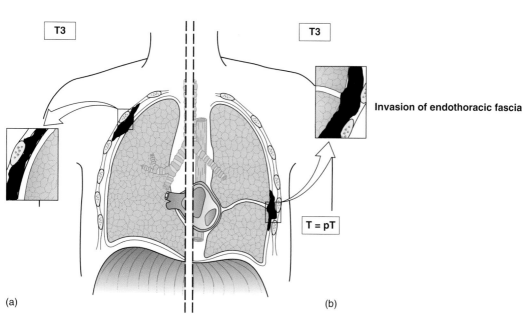

T3

T3

Invasion of endothoracic fascia

T = pT

(a)

(b)

Fig. 291

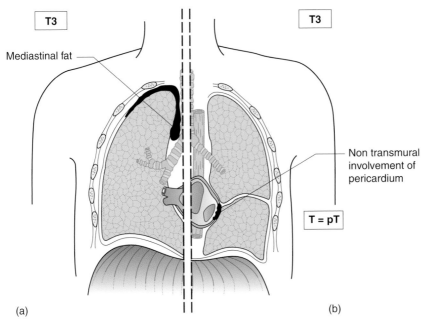

(a)   (b)

Fig. 292

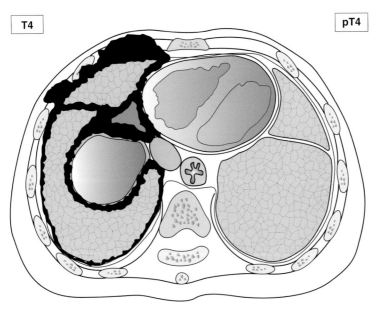

Fig. 293

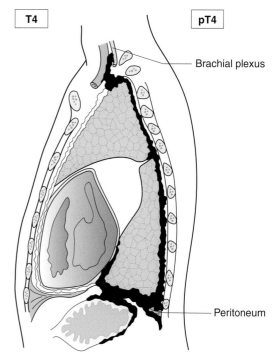

Fig. 294

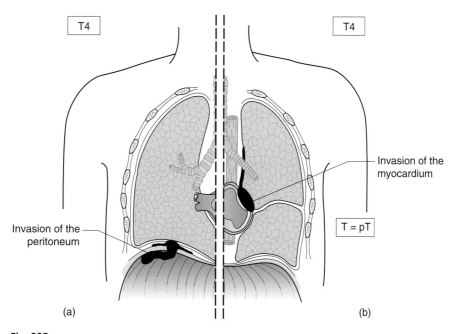

Fig. 295

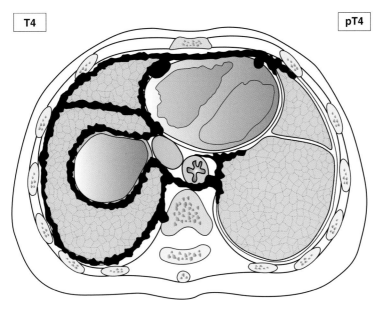

Fig. 296

N – Regional Lymph Nodes

NX   Regional lymph nodes cannot be assessed
N0   No regional lymph node metastasis
N1   Metastases to ipsilateral intrathoracic lymph nodes (includes ipsilateral bron-
      chopulmonary, hilar, subcarinal, paratracheal, aortopulmonary, paraesophageal,
      peridiaphragmatic, pericardial fat pad, intercostal and internal mammary nodes)
N2   Metastases to contralateral intrathoracic lymph nodes. Metastases to ipsilateral
      or contralateral supraclavicular lymph nodes

M – Distant Metastasis

M0   No distant metastasis
M1   Distant metastasis

pTNM Pathological Classification

The pT and pN categories correspond to the T and N categories.

pM1   Distant metastasis microscopically confirmed

Note
pM0 and pMX are not valid categories.

Summary

Pleural Mesothelioma

T1	Ipsilateral parietal pleura only with or without involvement of visceral, mediastinal, diaphragmatic pleura
T2	Invasion of ipsilateral diaphragmatic muscle and/or lung parenchyma
T3	Invasion of ipsilateral endothoracic fascia, mediastinal fat, focal chest wall, non-transmural pericardium
T4	Invasion of contralateral pleura, extensive chest wall, peritoneum, mediastinal organs, vertebra, neuroforamen, spinal cord, transmural pericardium, malignant pericardial effusion
N1	Ipsilateral intrathoracic (bronchopulmonary, hilar, subcarinal, paratracheal, aortopulmonary, paraesophageal, peridiaphragmatic, pericardial fat pad, intercostal, internal mammary)
N2	Contralateral intrathoracic, ipsilateral or contralateral supraclavicular
M1	Distant

Lung, pleural, thymic

THYMIC TUMOURS (ICD-0-3 C37.9)

Rules for Classification

The classification applies to epithelial tumours of the thymus, including thymomas, thymic carcinomas, and neuroendocrine tumours of the thymus. It does not apply to sarcomas, lymphomas and other rare tumours.

There should be histological confirmation of the disease and division of cases by histological type.

Regional Lymph Nodes

The regional lymph nodes for thymic tumours extend from the cervical region to the diaphragm. The lymph node mapping is performed according to the ITMIG/IASLC thymic nodal map.[1]

The regional lymph nodes are the anterior region (anterior mediastinal and anterior cervical) lymph nodes, the deep region (middle mediastinal lymph nodes and the deep cervical lymph nodes).

Notes
Clinical stage classification:
- The reliability of the imaging techniques in assessing involvement of the adjacent structures mostly relies on the radiologist's best judgement. Standard report terms for CT scan by ITMIG are available.[2]
- Any lymph node ≥ 1 cm in short axial dimension or with PET uptake (when available) should be considered involved for clinical staging and worth being removed at surgery.

Pathological stage classification:
- Specific attention should be paid by the surgeon to the intraoperative marking, orientation and handling of the surgical specimen. Also, standard report terms for the description of the surgical and pathological findings are encouraged. Recommendations by ITMIG for the handling of the surgical specimen and reporting of the surgical/pathological findings are available.[3]

[1] Bhora FY, Chen DJ, Detterbeck F. et al. (2014) The ITMIG/IASLC thymic epithelial tumors staging project: A proposed lymph node map for thymic epithelial tumors in the forthcoming 8th edition of the TNM classification of malignant tumors. *JTO* 9:S88–S96.

[2] Marom EM, Rosado-de-Christenson ML, Bruzzi JF, et al. (2011) Standard report terms for chest computed tomography reports of anterior mediastinal masses suspicious for thymoma. *JTO* 6:S1717–S1723.

[3] Detterbeck F, Moran C, Huang J, et al. (2011) Which way is up? Policies and procedures for surgeons and pathologists regarding resection specimens of thymic malignancy. *JTO* 7: S1730–S1738.

Correlation between clinical and pathological staging:

- Analysis of the literature indicates that the correlation between clinical and pathological stage in thymic epithelial tumours is only moderate, with more frequent upstaging than downstaging, particularly for thymic carcinoma.
- The most controversial areas are the involvement of major mediastinal structures, the identification of pleural/pericardial nodules and lymph nodal involvement.
- Although some imaging characteristics have been found to correlate either with the lack of invasion or the presence of invasion of mediastinal structures (Stage III), the reliability of these features is only moderate, with an error rate ranging from 20% up to 50%. Similarly, the reliability of identifying pleural/pericardial nodules (particularly if small), the involved lymph nodes (most are reactive) and the pulmonary nodules (the majority are benign) is limited.
- A detailed description of the CT findings predictive of invasiveness in thymoma is available.[4]

TNM Clinical Classification (cTNM)

T – Primary Tumour

TX   Primary tumour cannot be assessed

T0   No evidence of primary tumour

T1   Tumour encapsulated or extending into the mediastinal fat, may involve the mediastinal pleura

   T1a   No mediastinal pleura involvement

   T1b   Direct invasion of the mediastinal pleura

T2   Tumour with direct involvement of the pericardium (partial or full thickness)

T3   Tumour with direct invasion into any of the following:
- Lung
- Brachiocephalic vein
- Superior vena cava
- Phrenic nerve
- Chest wall
- Extrapericardial pulmonary artery or vein.

T4   Tumour with direct invasion into any of the following:
- Aorta (ascending, arch, or descending)
- Arch vessels
- Intrapericardial pulmonary artery or vein
- Myocardium
- Trachea
- Oesophagus

[4] Marom E, Milito M, Moran C, et al. (2011) Computed tomography findings predicting invasiveness of thymoma. *JTO* 6(7):1274–1281.

Notes
- For pathologic T classification involvement of any structure should be microscopically confirmed. Adhesion of the tumour to an adjacent structure identified by the surgeon should not be considered for the T classification.
- The T category is determined by the level of involvement. The T category is assigned to the highest level of involvement, regardless of involvement of structures of a lower level.
- Direct invasion of the lung and the pleura is assigned to the T category and should be distinguished from separated lung and pleural nodules (see M category).

N – Regional Lymph Nodes

NX   Regional lymph nodes cannot be assessed
N0   No regional lymph node metastasis
N1   Metastasis in anterior (perithymic) lymph nodes
N2   Metastasis in deep intrathoracic or deep cervical lymph nodes

Notes
- Direct extension of the primary tumour into a lymph node is considered as nodal involvement.
- Lymph node dissection or sampling during resection of thymic tumours is strongly recommended, and the pathologists should specifically examine and report on the presence of nodal involvement. ITMIG/IASLC recommendations for lymph node dissection are as follows:
  - Any suspicious lymph node at surgery or at preoperative imaging should be removed.
  - For T1–T2 thymomas removal of adjacent nodes and anterior mediastinal nodes.
  - For >T2 thymomas systematic anterior mediastinal node dissection and sampling of deep mediastinal appropriate areas (paratracheal, aortopulmonary).
  - For thymic carcinomas a systematic sampling of N1 and N2 regions according to the ITMIG/IASLC nodal map (anterior mediastinal, intrathoracic, supraclavicular and lower cervical lymph nodes).

M – Distant Metastasis

M0   No pleural, pericardial or distant metastasis
M1   Distant metastasis
      M1a Separate pleural or pericardial nodule(s)
      M1b Distant metastasis beyond the pleura or pericardium, including separate pulmonary nodules

Notes
- Pleural or pericardial nodes that are completely separated from the primary tumour are to be classified as M1a.
- Lung nodules that are surrounded by normal parenchyma (and not in direct extension to the primary tumour) are to be classified as M1b.

TNM Pathological Classification (pTNM)

The pT, and pN categories correspond to the T and N categories.
  pM1 Distant metastasis microscopically confirmed

Note
pM0 and pMX are not valid categories.

Stage Grouping

Stage I (Figs. 297, 298)	T1a	N0	M0
	T1b		
Stage II (Fig. 299)	T2	N0	M0
Stage IIIA (Fig. 300)	T3	N0	M0
Stage IIIB (Fig. 301)	T4	N0	M0
Stage IVA (Fig. 302)	Any T	N1	M0
	Any T	N0, N1	M1a
Stage IVB (Fig. 303)	Any T	N2	M0, M1a
	Any T	Any N	M1b

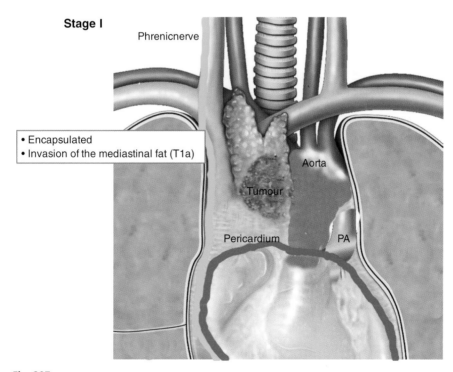

Stage I

Phrenicnerve

• Encapsulated
• Invasion of the mediastinal fat (T1a)

Aorta

Tumour

Pericardium   PA

Fig. 297

Stage I

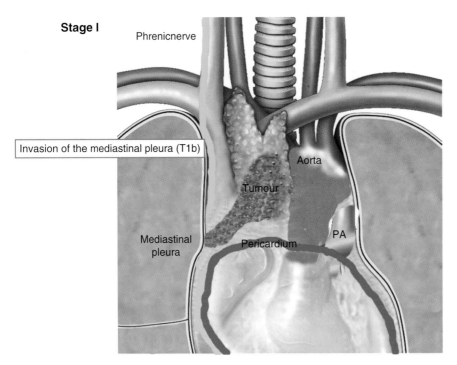

Phrenicnerve

Invasion of the mediastinal pleura (T1b)

Aorta

Tumour

Mediastinal
pleura

Pericardium

PA

Fig. 298

Stage II

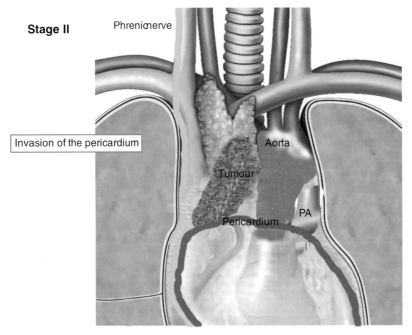

Phrenicnerve

Invasion of the pericardium

Aorta

Tumour

Pericardium

PA

Fig. 299

Stage IIIA

Phrenic nerve

Invasion of one of the following:
- Lung
- Phrenic nerve
- Brachiocephalicvein
- Superiorvena cava
- Extrapericardial PA and PV
- Chestwall

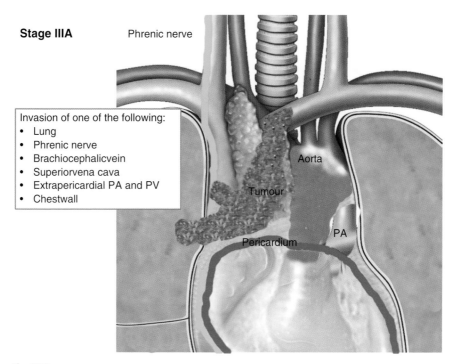

Fig. 300

Stage IIIB

Phrenicnerve

Invasion of one of the following:
- Aorta
- Arch vessels
- Myocardium
- Intrapericardial PA and PV
- Trachea
- Oesophagus

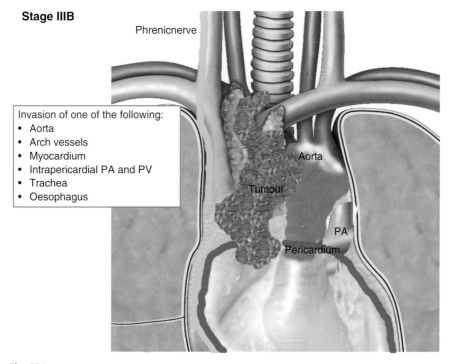

Fig. 301

Stage IVA

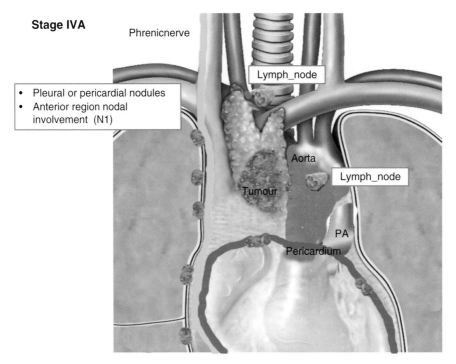

- Pleural or pericardial nodules
- Anterior region nodal involvement (N1)

Fig. 302

Stage IVB

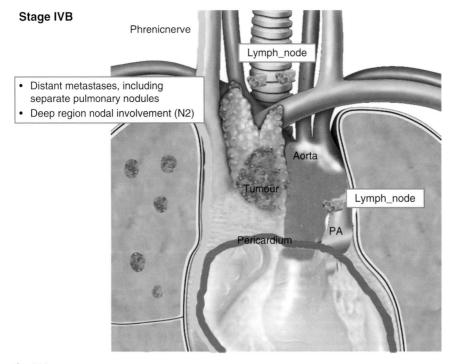

- Distant metastases, including separate pulmonary nodules
- Deep region nodal involvement (N2)

Fig. 303

Summary

TX	Primary tumour cannot be assessed
T0	No evidence of primary tumour
T1	Tumour encapsulated or extending into the mediastinal fat, may involve the mediastinal pleura
	T1a No mediastinal pleura involvement
	T1b Direct invasion of the mediastinal pleura
T2	Tumour with direct involvement of the pericardium (partial or full thickness)
T3	Tumour with direct invasion into any of the following: lung; brachiocephalic vein; superior vena cava; phrenic nerve; chest wall; extrapericardial pulmonary artery or vein
T4	Tumour with direct invasion into any of the following: aorta (ascending, arch or descending); arch vessels; intrapericardial pulmonary artery or vein; myocardium; trachea; oesophagus
NX	Regional lymph nodes cannot be assessed
N0	No regional lymph node metastasis
N1	Metastasis in anterior (perithymic) lymph nodes
N2	Metastasis in deep intrathoracic or deep cervical lymph nodes
M0	No pleural, pericardial or distant metastasis
M1	Distant metastasis
	M1a Separate pleural or pericardial nodule(s)
	M1b Distant metastasis beyond the pleura or pericardium

The ITMIG/IASLC thymic nodal map

Anterior region (N1): Anterior mediastinal and anterior cervical nodes

Region Boundaries	Node Groups	Node Group Boundaries
Sup: Hyoid Bone Lat (Neck): Medial Border of Carotid Sheaths Lat (Chest): Mediastinal Pleura Ant: Sternum Post (Medially): Great Vessels, Pericardium Post (Laterally): Phrenic Nerve Inf: Xiphoid, diaphragm	Low Ant Cervical: Pretracheal, Paratracheal, Peri-thyroid, Precricoid/ Delphian (AAO-HNS / ASHNS Level 6 / IASLC Level 1)	Sup: inferior border of cricoid Lat: common carotid arteries Inf: superior border of manubrium
	Peri-Thymic	Proximity to thymus
	Pre vascular(IASLC Level 3a)	Sup: apex of chest Ant: posterior sternum Post: anterior SVC Inf: carina
	Paraaortic, Ascending Aorta, Superior Phrenics (IASLC Level 6)	Sup: line tangential to sup border of aortic arch Inf: inf border of aortic arch
	Supradiaphragmatic / Inferior Phrenics / Pericardial (along inferior poles of thymus)	Sup: inf border of aortic arch Ant: post sternum Post: phrenic nerve (laterally) or pericardium (medially) Inf: diaphragm

Deep region (N2): Middle mediastinum and deep cervical nodes (+ internal mammary nodes)

Region Boundaries	Node Groups	Node Group Boundaries
Sup; Level of lower border of cricoid cartilage Anteromedial (Neck): Lateral Border of Sternohyoid, Medial Border of Carotid Sheath Posterolateral (Neck): Anterior Border of Trapezius Ant (Chest): Aortic Arch, Aortopulmonary Window – Ant Border of SVC Post (Chest): Esophagus Lat (Chest): Pulmonary Hila Inf: Diaphragm	Lower Jugular (AAO-HNS / ASHNS Level 4)	Sup: Level of lower border of cricoid cartilage Anteromedial: lat border of sternohyoid Posterolateral: lat border of sternocleidomastoid Inf: clavicle
	Supraclavicular/Venous Angle: Confluence of Internal Jugular & Subclavian Vein (AAO-HNS / ASHNS Level 5b)	Sup: Level of lower border of cricoid cartilage Anteromedial; post border of sternocleidomastoid Posterolateral: ant border of trapezius Inf: clavicle
	Internal Mammary nodes	Proximity to internal mammary arteries
	Upper Paratracheal (IASLC Level 2)	Sup: sup border of manubrium, apices of lungs Inf: intersection of lower border of innominate vein with trachea; sup border of aortic arch
	Lower Paratracheal (IASLC Level 4)	Sup: intersection of lower border of innominate vein with trachea; sup border of aortic arch Inf: lower border of azygos vein, sup border of left main pulmonary artery
	Subaortic / Aortopulmonary Window (IASLC Level 5)	Sup: inf border of aortic arch Inf: sup border of left main pulmonary artery
	Subcarinal (IASLC Level 7)	Sup: carina Inf: upper border of lower lobe bronchus on the left; lower border of the bronchus intermedius on the right
	Hilar (IASLC Level LO)	Sup: lower rim of azygos vein on right, upper rim of pulmonary artery on left Inf: interlobar region bilaterally

BONE AND SOFT TISSUE TUMOURS

Introductory Notes

The following sites are included:
- Bone
- Soft tissues
- Gastrointestinal stromal tumours

G Histopathological Grading

The staging of bone and soft tissue sarcomas is based on a three-tiered grade classification. In this classification, Grade 1 is considered "low grade" and Grades 2 and 3 "high grade".

Regional Lymph Nodes

The regional lymph nodes are those appropriate to the site of the primary tumour. Regional node metastases are rare.

The definitions of the N categories for all tumours of bone and soft tissues are as follows.

N – Regional Lymph Nodes

NX   Regional lymph nodes cannot be assessed
N0   No regional lymph node metastasis
N1   Regional lymph node metastasis

TNM Atlas: Illustrated Guide to the TNM Classification of Malignant Tumours, Seventh Edition.
Edited by James D. Brierley, Hisao Asamura, Elisabeth Van Eycken, and Brian Rous.
© 2021 by UICC. Published 2021 by John Wiley & Sons Ltd.

BONE (ICD-O-3 C40, 41)

Rules for Classification

The classification applies to all primary malignant bone tumours except malignant lymphomas, multiple myeloma, surface/juxtacortical osteosarcoma and juxtacortical chondrosarcoma. There should be histological confirmation of the disease and division of cases by histological type and grade.

TNM Clinical Classification

T – Primary Tumour

TX   Primary tumour cannot be assessed
T0   No evidence of primary tumour

Appendicular Skeleton, Trunk, Skull and Facial Bones

T1   Tumour 8 cm or less in greatest dimension (Fig. 304, 305)
T2   Tumour more than 8 cm in greatest dimension (Fig. 306, 307)
T3   Discontinuous tumours in the primary bone site (Fig. 308)

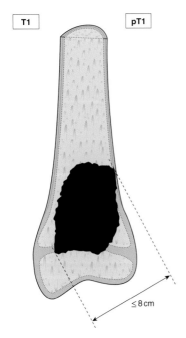

T1   pT1

≤8 cm

Fig. 304

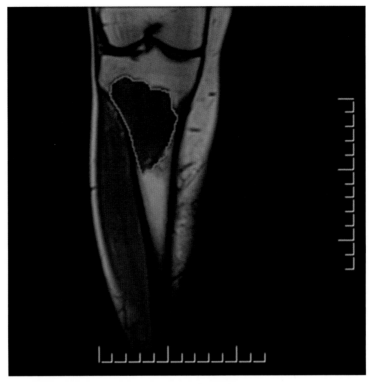

Fig. 305   T1 sarcoma of the tibia 8 cm in greatest dimension

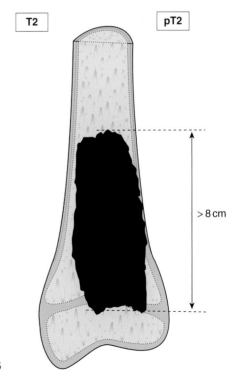

Fig. 306

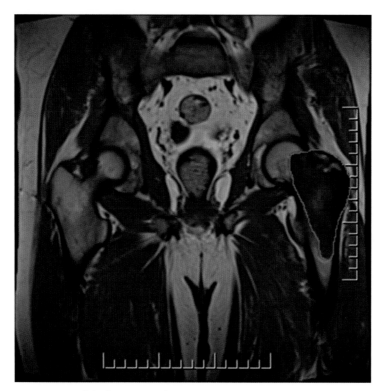

Fig. 307   T2 sarcoma of the femur more than 8 cm in greatest dimension (14 cm)

T3   pT3

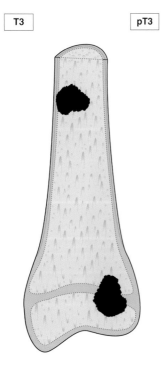

Fig. 308

Spine

T1   Tumour confined to a single vertebral segment or two adjacent vertebral segments

T2   Tumour confined to three adjacent vertebral segments

T3   Tumour confined to four adjacent vertebral segments

T4a   Tumour invades into the spinal canal

T4b   Tumour invades the adjacent vessels or tumour thrombosis within the adjacent vessels

Note

The five vertebral segments (Fig. 309) are:

- Right pedicle
- Right body
- Left body
- Left pedicle
- Posterior element

Pelvis

T1a   A tumour no more than 8 cm in size and confined to a single pelvic segment with no extraosseous extension

T1b   A tumour greater than 8 cm in size and confined to a single pelvic segment with no extraosseous extension

T2a   A tumour no more than 8 cm in size and confined to a single pelvic segment with extraosseous extension or confined to two adjacent pelvic segments without extraosseous extension

T2b   A tumour greater than 8 cm in size and confined to a single pelvic segment with extraosseous extension or confined to two adjacent pelvic segments without extraosseous extension

T3a   A tumour no more than 8 cm in size and confined to two pelvic segments with extraosseous extension

T3b   A tumour greater than 8 cm in size and confined to two pelvic segments with extraosseous extension

T4a   Tumour involving three adjacent pelvic segments or crossing the sacroiliac joint to the sacral neuroforamen

T4b   Tumour encasing the external iliac vessels or gross tumour thrombus in major pelvic vessels

Note

The four pelvic segments (Fig. 310) are:

- Sacrum lateral to sacral foramen
- Iliac wing
- Acetabulum/periacetabulum
- Pelvic rami, symphysis and ischium

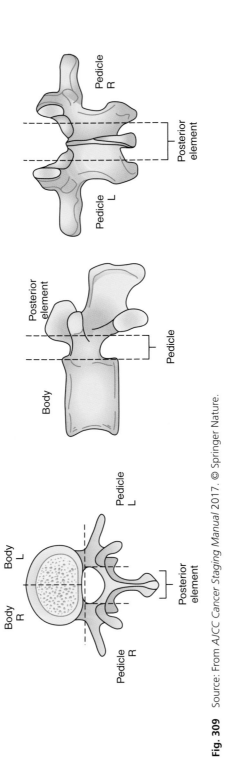

Fig. 309 Source: From *AJCC Cancer Staging Manual* 2017. © Springer Nature.

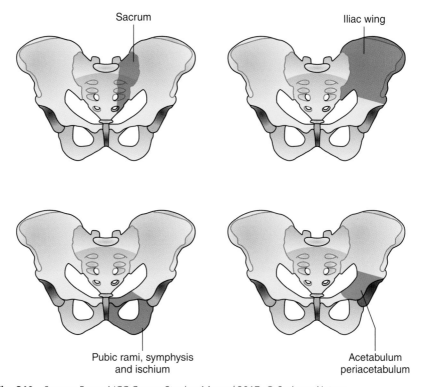

Fig. 310 Source: From *AJCC Cancer Staging Manual* 2017. © Springer Nature.

N – Regional Lymph Nodes

NX   Regional lymph nodes cannot be assessed
N0   No regional lymph node metastasis
N1   Regional lymph node metastasis

M – Distant Metastasis

M0   No distant metastasis
M1   Distant metastasis
    M1a   Lung
    M1b   Other distant sites

pTNM Pathological Classification

The pT and pN categories correspond to the T and N categories.

pM1   Distant metastasis microscopically confirmed

Note
pM0 and pMX are not valid categories.

Summary

Appendicular Skeleton, Trunk, Skull and Facial Bones	
T1	≤ 8 cm
T2	> 8 cm
T3	Discontinuous tumours in primary site
Spine	
T1	Single or 2 adjacent segments
T2	3 adjacent segments
T3	4 adjacent segments
T4a	Into spinal canal
T4b	Into adjacent vessels or tumour thrombus in adjacent vessels
Pelvis	
T1a	≤ 8 cm confined to single segment
T1b	> 8 cm confined to single segment
T2a	≤ 8 cm confined to single segment with extraosseous extension or
	≤ 8 cm confined to two segments without extension
T2b	> 8 cm confined to single segment with extraosseous extension or
	> 8 cm confined to two segments without extension
T3a	≤ 8 cm confined to two segments with extraosseous extension or
T3b	> 8 cm confined to single segment with extraosseous extension
T4a	Three segments or crossing SI joint into foramen
T4b	Encasing external iliac vessels or tumour thrombus in major pelvic vessels
N1	Regional
M1a	Lung
M1b	Other sites

SOFT TISSUES (ICD-O-3 C38.1–3, C47–49)

Rules for Classification

There should be histological confirmation of the disease and division of cases by histological type and grade.

Anatomical Sites

1. Connective, subcutaneous, and other soft tissues (C49), peripheral nerves (C47)
2. Retroperitoneum (C48.0)
3. Mediastinum: anterior (38.1); posterior (C38.2); mediastinum, NOS (C38.3)

Histological Types of Tumour

The following histological types are not included:
- Kaposi sarcoma
- Dermatofibrosarcoma (protuberans)
- Fibromatosis (desmoid tumour)
- Sarcoma arising from the dura mater or brain
- Angiosarcoma, an aggressive sarcoma, is excluded because its natural history is not consistent with the classification

Note
Cystosarcoma phylloides is staged as a soft tissue sarcoma of the superficial trunk.

Regional Lymph Nodes

The regional lymph nodes are those appropriate to the site of the primary tumour. Regional node involvement is rare, and cases in which nodal status is not assessed either clinically or pathologically could be considered N0 instead of NX or pNX.

TNM Clinical Classification

T – Primary Tumour – Extremity and Superficial Trunk

TX   Primary tumour cannot be assessed
T0   No evidence of primary tumour

T1   Tumour 5 cm or less in greatest dimension (Figs. 311, 312)

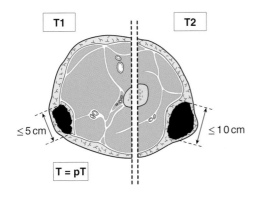

Fig. 311

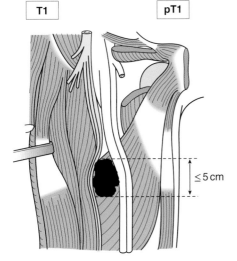

Fig. 312

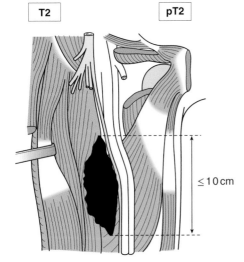

Fig. 313

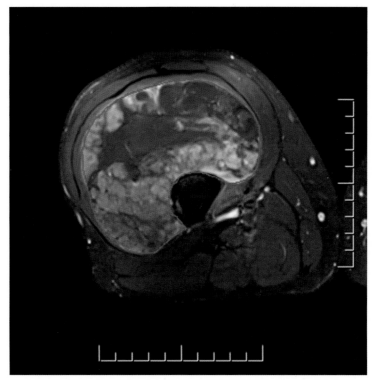

Fig. 314   T3 sarcoma 12 cm in greatest dimension.

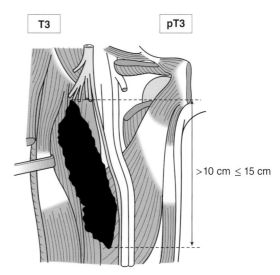

Fig. 315

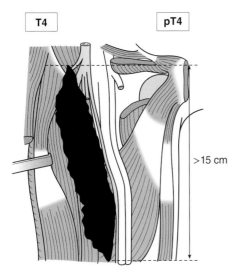

>15 cm

Fig. 316

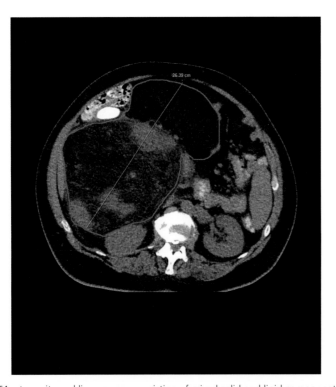

Fig. 317   T4 retroperitoneal liposarcoma consisting of mixed solid and lipid components measuring 26.5 cm in greatest dimension.

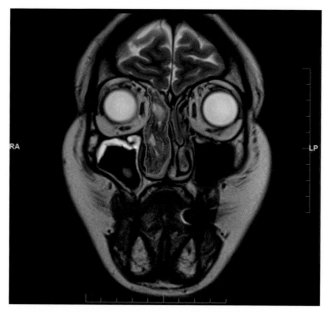

Fig. 318 Low grade sinonasal sarcoma T3 in greatest dimension.

T2   Tumour more than 5 cm but no more than 10 cm in greatest dimension (Figs. 311, 313)

T3   Tumour more than 10 cm but no more than 15 cm in greatest dimension (Fig. 314)

T4   Tumour more than 15 cm in greatest dimension (Fig. 315, 316)

Retroperitoneum

T1   Tumour 5 cm or less in greatest dimension

T2   Tumour more than 5 cm but no more than 10 cm in greatest dimension (Fig. 316)

T3   Tumour more than 10 cm but no more than 15 cm in greatest dimension

T4   Tumour more than 15 cm in greatest dimension (Fig. 317)

Head and Neck

T1   Tumour 2 cm or less in greatest dimension

T2   Tumour more than 2 cm but no more than 4 cm in greatest

T3   Tumour more than 4 cm in greatest dimension (Fig. 318)

T4a   Tumour invades the orbit, skull base or dura, central compartment viscera, facial skeleton and/or pterygoid muscles

T4b   Tumour invades the brain parenchyma, encases the carotid artery, invades prevertebral muscle or involves the central nervous system by perineural spread

Thoracic and Abdominal Viscera

T1	Tumour confined to a single organ
T2a	Tumour invades serosa or visceral peritoneum
T2b	Tumour with microscopic extension beyond the serosa
T3	Tumour invades another organ or macroscopic extension beyond the serosa
T4a	Multifocal tumour involving no more than 2 sites in one organ
T4b	Multifocal tumour involving more than 2 sites but not more than 5 sites
T4c	Multifocal tumour involving more than 5 sites

N – Regional Lymph Nodes

NX	Regional lymph nodes cannot be assessed
N0	No regional lymph node metastasis
N1	Regional lymph node metastasis

M – Distant Metastasis

M0	No distant metastasis
M1	Distant metastasis

pTNM Pathological Classification

The pT and pN categories correspond to the T and N categories.

pM1   Distant metastasis microscopically confirmed

Note
pM0 and pMX are not valid categories.

GASTROINTESTINAL STROMAL TUMOURS (GIST)

Rules for Classification

The classification applies only to gastrointestinal stromal tumours. There should be histological confirmation of the disease.

Anatomical Sites and Subsites

- Oesophagus (C15)
- Stomach (C16)
- Small intestine (C17)
  1. Duodenum (C17.0)
  2. Jejunum (C17.1)
  3. Ileum (C17.2)
- Colon (C18)
- Rectum (C20)
- Omentum (C48.1)
- Mesentery (C48.1)

Regional Lymph Nodes

The regional lymph nodes are those appropriate to the site of the primary tumour; see gastrointestinal sites for details.

TNM Clinical Classification

T – Primary Tumour

TX	Primary tumour cannot be assessed
T0	No evidence for primary tumour
T1	Tumour 2 cm or less in greater dimension (Fig. 319)
T2	Tumour more than 2 cm but not more than 5 cm (Fig. 319)
T3	Tumour more than 5 cm but not more than 10 cm (Fig. 320)
T4	Tumour more than 10 cm in greatest dimension (Fig. 320)

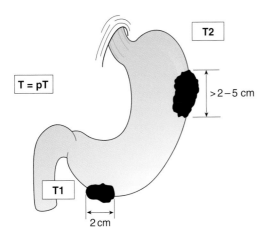

T2

T = pT

>2–5 cm

T1

2 cm

Fig. 319

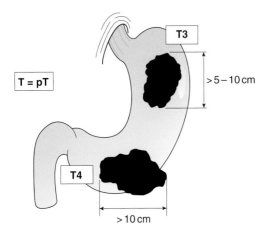

T3

T = pT

>5–10 cm

T4

>10 cm

Fig. 320

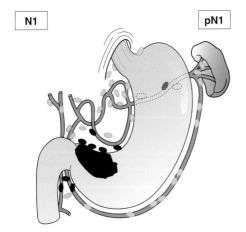

N1

pN1

Fig. 321

N – Regional Lymph Nodes

NX   Regional lymph nodes cannot be assessed*
N0   No regional lymph node metastasis
N1   Regional lymph node metastasis (Fig. 321)

Note
*NX: Regional lymph node involvement is rare for GISTs, so that cases in which the nodal status is not assessed clinically or pathologically could be considered N0 instead of NX or pNX.

M – Distant Metastasis

M0   No distant metastasis
M1   Distant metastasis

pTNM Pathological Classification

The pT and pN categories correspond to the T and N categories.

pM1   Distant metastasis microscopically confirmed

Note
pM0 and pMX are not valid categories.

G Histopathological Grading

Grading for GIST is dependent on mitotic rate.*
    Low mitotic rate: 5 or fewer per 50 hpf
    High mitotic rate: over 5 per 50 hpf

Note
*The mitotic rate of GIST is best expressed as the number of mitoses per 50 high power fields (hpf) using the 40× objective (total area 5 mm^2 in 50 fields).

Summary

Gastrointestinal Stromal Tumour	
T1	≤ 2 cm
T2	> 2–5 cm
T3	> 5–10 cm
T4	> 10 cm
N1	Regional
M1	Distant metastasis

SKIN TUMOURS

Introductory Notes

The classifications apply to carcinomas of the skin, [excluding vulva (see Gynaecological Tumours), and penis (see Urological Tumours), and perianal skin (see Gastrointestinal Tumours)], to malignant melanomas of the skin including eyelid and to Merkel cell carcinoma.

Anatomical Sites

The following sites are identified by ICD-O-3 topography rubrics:
- Lip (excluding vermilion surface) (C44.0)
- Eyelid (C44.1)
- External ear (C44.2)
- Other and unspecified parts of face (C44.3)
- Scalp and neck (C44.4)
- Trunk excluding anal margin and perianal skin (C44.5)
- Upper limb and shoulder (C44.6)
- Lower limb and hip (C44.7)
- Scrotum (C63.2)

TNM Atlas: Illustrated Guide to the TNM Classification of Malignant Tumours, Seventh Edition.
Edited by James D. Brierley, Hisao Asamura, Elisabeth Van Eycken, and Brian Rous.
© 2021 by UICC. Published 2021 by John Wiley & Sons Ltd.

Regional Lymph Nodes (Figs. 322, 323)

The regional lymph nodes are those appropriate to the site of the primary tumour.

Unilateral Tumours

- **Head, neck**: Ipsilateral preauricular, submandibular, cervical, and supraclavicular lymph nodes
- **Thorax**: Ipsilateral axillary lymph nodes
- **Upper limb**: Ipsilateral epitrochlear and axillary lymph nodes
- **Abdomen, loins, and buttocks**: Ipsilateral inguinal lymph nodes
- **Lower limb**: Ipsilateral popliteal and inguinal lymph nodes
- **Anal margin and perianal skin**: Ipsilateral inguinal lymph nodes

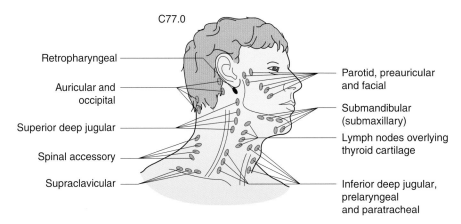

Fig. 322

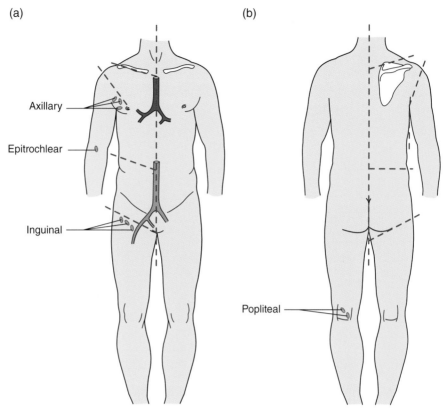

Fig. 323

Tumours in the Boundary Zones between the Above

The lymph nodes pertaining to the regions on both sides of the boundary zone are considered to be the regional lymph nodes.

The following 4-cm-wide bands are considered as boundary zones (Figs. 323, 324, 325, 326, 327, 328).

Between	*Along*
Right/left	Midline
Head and neck/thorax	Clavicula-acromion-upper shoulder blade edge
Thorax/upper limb	Shoulder-axilla-shoulder
Thorax/abdomen, loins, and buttocks	*Front*: middle between navel and costal arch
	Back: lower border of thoracic vertebrae (midtransverse axis)
Abdomen, loins, and buttock/ lower limb	Groin-trochanter-gluteal sulcus

Any metastasis to other than the listed regional lymph nodes is considered as M1 (Figs. 324, 325, 326, 327, 328).

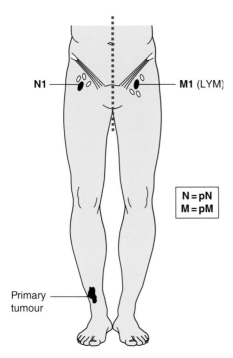

N1

M1 (LYM)

N = pN
M = pM

Primary
tumour

Fig. 324

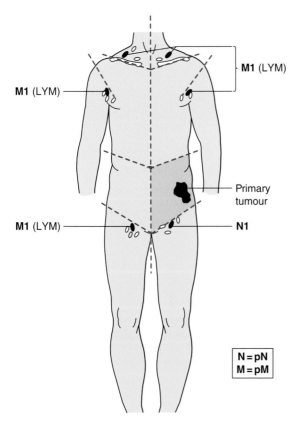

M1 (LYM)

M1 (LYM)

M1 (LYM)

M1 (LYM)

Primary
tumour

N1

N = pN
M = pM

Fig. 325

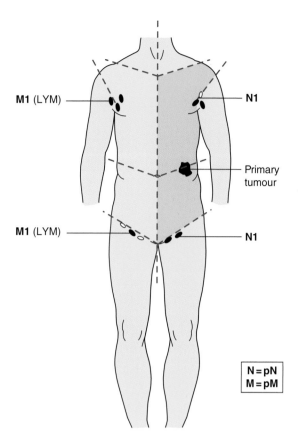

Fig. 326

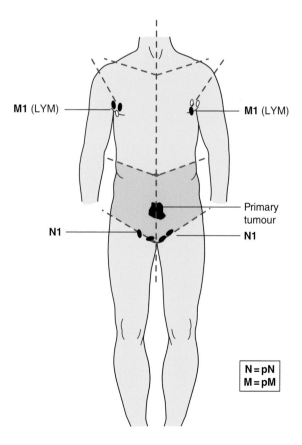

Fig. 327

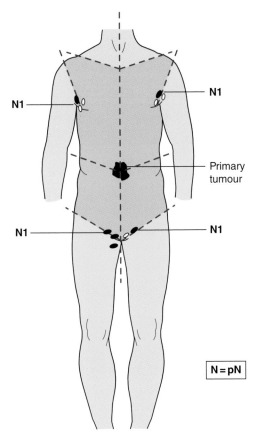

N1

N1

Primary
tumour

N1

N1

N = pN

Fig. 328

CARCINOMA OF THE SKIN (EXCLUDING EYELID, HEAD AND NECK, PERIANAL, VULVA, AND PENIS) (ICD-O-3 C44.5–7, C63.2)

Rules for Classification

The classification applies only to carcinomas, excluding Merkel cell carcinoma. There should be histological confirmation of the disease and division of cases by histological type.

Regional Lymph Nodes

The regional lymph nodes are those appropriate to the site of the primary tumour. See Regional Lymph Nodes under Skin Tumours.

TNM Clinical Classification

T – Primary Tumour

TX   Primary tumour cannot be assessed
T0   No evidence of primary tumour
Tis   Carcinoma in situ (Fig. 329)

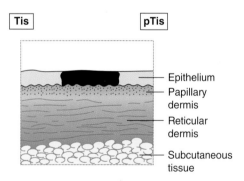

Fig. 329

T1   Tumour 2 cm or less in greatest dimension (Fig. 330)
T2   Tumour > 2 cm and ≤ 4 cm in greatest dimension (Fig. 331)
T3   Tumour > 4 cm in maximum dimension or minor bone erosion or perineural inva-
      sion or deep invasion* (Fig. 332)
T4a   Tumour with gross cortical bone/ marrow invasion,
T4b   Tumour with axial skeleton invasion including foraminal involvement and/or ver-
      tebral foramen involvement to the epidural space.

*Deep invasion is defined as invasion beyond the subcutaneous fat or > 6 mm (as measured from
the granular layer of adjacent normal epidermis to the base of the tumour), perineural invasion for
T3 classification is defined as clinical or radiographic involvement of named nerves without foramen
or skull base invasion or transgression.

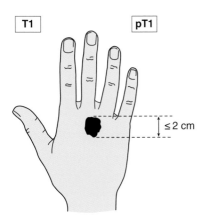

Fig. 330

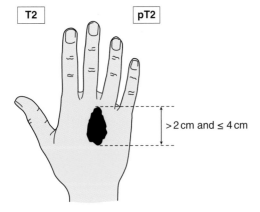

Fig. 331

Skin

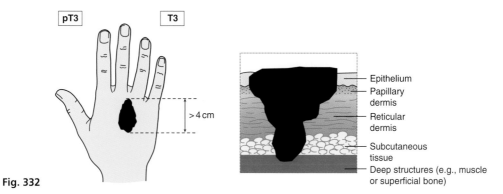

Fig. 332

Note

In the case of multiple simultaneous tumours, the tumour with the highest T category is classified and the number of separate tumours is indicated in parentheses, e.g., T2(5) (Fig. 333)

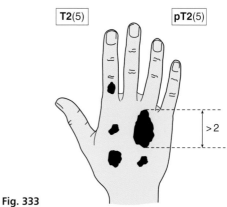

Fig. 333

N – Regional Lymph Nodes

NX   Regional lymph nodes cannot be assessed

N0   No regional lymph node metastasis

N1   Metastasis in a single ipsilateral lymph node, 3 cm or less in greatest dimension

N2   Metastasis in a single ipsilateral lymph node, more than 3 cm but not more than 6 cm in greatest dimension, or in multiple ipsilateral lymph nodes, none more than 6 cm in greatest dimension, or in bilateral or contralateral lymph nodes, none more than 6 cm in greatest dimension

N3   Metastasis in a lymph node, more than 6 cm in greatest dimension

M – Distant Metastasis

M0   No distant metastasis

M1   Distant metastasis (Figs. 324, 325, 326, 327, 328)

pTNM Pathological Classification

The pT, and pN categories correspond to the T and N categories.

pM1   Distant metastasis microscopically confirmed

Note

pM0 and pMX are not valid categories.

pN0   Histological examination of a regional lymphadenectomy specimen will ordinarily include 6 or more lymph nodes. If the lymph nodes are negative, but the number ordinarily examined is not met, classify as pN0.

Summary

Skin Carcinoma	
T1	≤ 2 cm
T2	> 2 cm and ≤ 4 cm
T3	> 4 cm or deep structures
T4a	Bone invasion
T4b	Axial skeleton
N1	Ipsilateral single, ≤ 3 cm
N2	Ipsilateral single, > 3 to 6 cm
	Ipsilateral multiple, ≤ 6 cm
	Bilateral, contralateral, ≤ 6 cm
N3	> 6 cm
M1	Distant

CARCINOMA OF SKIN OF THE HEAD AND NECK (ICD-O-3 C44.0, C44.2–4)

Rules for Classification

The classification applies only to carcinomas, excluding Merkel cell carcinoma. There should be histological confirmation of the disease and division of cases by histological type.

Anatomical Sites and Subsites

The following sites are identified by ICD-O-3 topography rubrics (see Fig. 334):
- Lip (excluding vermilion surface) (C44.0)
- External ear (C44.2)
- Other and unspecified parts of face (C44.3)
- Scalp and neck (C44.4)

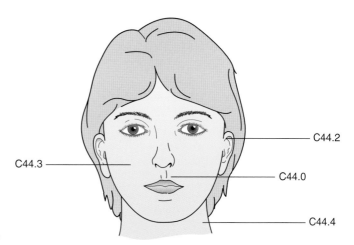

C44.2

C44.3

C44.0

C44.4

Fig. 334

Regional Lymph Nodes

The regional lymph nodes are Ipsilateral preauricular, submandibular, cervical and supra-clavicular lymph nodes (see Fig. 335).

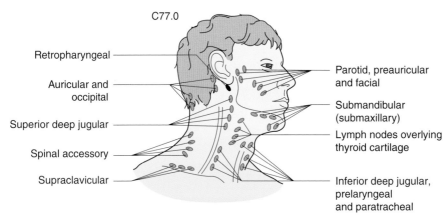

Fig. 335

TNM Clinical Classification

T – Primary Tumour

Tx   Primary tumour cannot be assessed
T0   No evidence of primary tumour
Tis   Carcinoma in situ (Fig. 336)

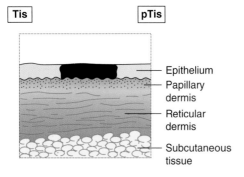

Fig. 336

T1	Tumour 2 cm or less in greatest dimension (Fig. 337)
T2	Tumour > 2 cm and ≤ 4 cm in greatest dimension (Fig. 338)
T3	Tumour > 4 cm in maximum dimension or minor bone erosion or perineural invasion or deep invasion* (Fig. 339)
T4a	Tumour with gross cortical bone/marrow invasion
T4b	Tumour with skull base or axial skeleton invasion including foraminal involvement and/or vertebral foramen involvement to the epidural space

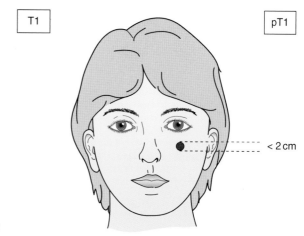

Fig. 337

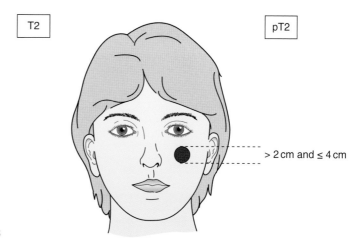

Fig. 338

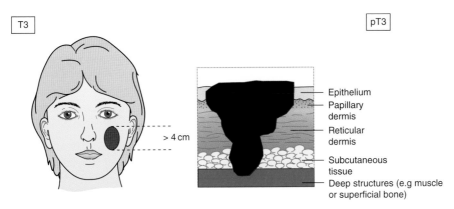

Fig. 339

Note

*In the case of multiple simultaneous tumours, the tumour with the highest T category is classified and the number of separate tumours is indicated in parentheses, e.g., T2(5) (Fig. 340)

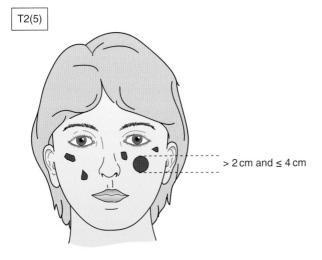

Fig. 340

N – Regional Lymph Nodes

N0   No regional lymph node metastasis

N1   Metastasis in a single ipsilateral lymph node, 3 cm or less in greatest dimension without extranodal extension (Fig. 341)

N2   Metastasis as described below:

    N2a   Metastasis in a single ipsilateral lymph node more than 3 cm but not more than 6 cm in greatest dimension without extranodal extension (Fig. 342)

N2b   Metastasis in multiple ipsilateral lymph nodes, none more than 6 cm in greatest dimension, without extranodal extension (Fig. 343)

N2c   Metastasis in bilateral or contralateral lymph nodes, none more than 6 cm in greatest dimension, without extranodal extension (Fig. 344)

N3a   Metastasis in a lymph node more than 6 cm in greatest dimension without extranodal extension (Fig. 345)

N3b   Metastasis in single or multiple lymph nodes with clinical extranodal extension

Note

*The presence of skin involvement or soft tissue invasion with deep fixation/tethering to underlying muscle or adjacent structures or clinical signs of nerve involvement is classified as clinical extranodal extension.

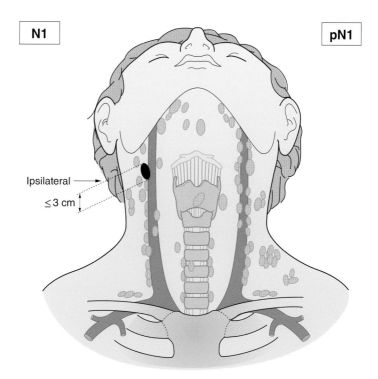

Fig. 341

N2a

pN2a

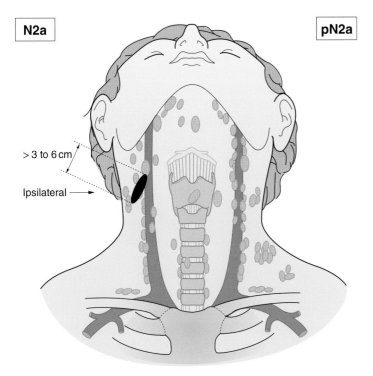

> 3 to 6 cm

Ipsilateral

Fig. 342

Skin

N2b

pN2b

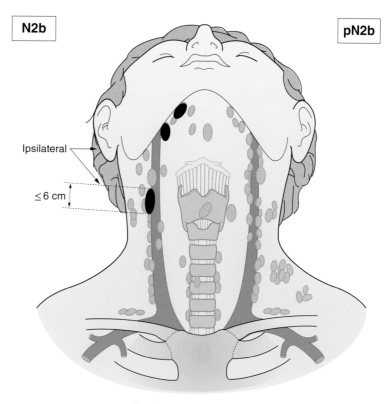

Ipsilateral

≤ 6 cm

Fig. 343

N2c

pN2c

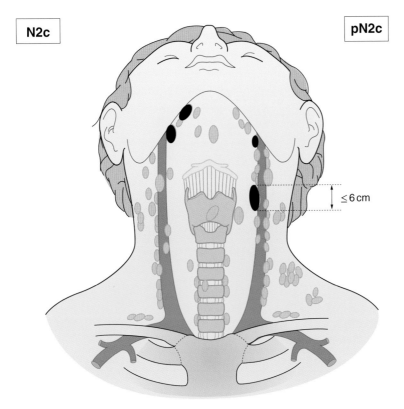

≤ 6 cm

Fig. 344

N3a

pN3a

Skin

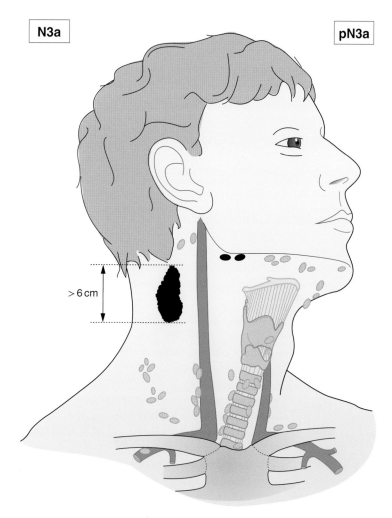

> 6 cm

Fig. 345

M – Distant Metastasis

M0   No distant metastasis
M1   Distant metastasis

pTNM Pathological Classification

The pT categories correspond to the T categories.

pN – Regional Lymph Nodes

Histological examination of a selective neck dissection specimen will ordinarily include 10 or more lymph nodes. Histological examination of a radical or modified radical neck dissection specimen will ordinarily include 15 or more lymph nodes.

pNX   Regional lymph nodes cannot be assessed
pN0   No regional lymph node metastasis
pN1   Metastasis in a single ipsilateral lymph node, 3 cm or less in greatest dimension without extranodal extension
pN2   Metastasis as described below:
    pN2a   Metastasis in a single ipsilateral lymph node, less than 3 cm in greatest dimension with extranodal extension, or more than 3 cm but not more than 6 cm in greatest dimension without extranodal extension
    pN2b   Metastasis in multiple ipsilateral lymph nodes, none more than 6 cm in greatest dimension without extranodal extension
    pN2c   Metastasis in bilateral or contralateral lymph nodes, none more than 6 cm in greatest dimension without extranodal extension
pN3a   Metastasis in a lymph node more than 6 cm in greatest dimension without extranodal extension
pN3b   Metastasis in a lymph node more than 3 cm in greatest dimension with extranodal extension, or multiple ipsilateral, contralateral or bilateral, with extranodal extension

pM – Distant metastasis

pM1   Distant metastasis microscopically confirmed

Note
pM0 and pMx are not categories.

Summary

Skin Carcinoma of the Head and Neck

T1	≤ 2 cm
T2	> 2 cm and ≤ 4 cm
T3	> 4 cm or deep structures
T4a	Bone invasion
T4b	Axial skeleton
N1	Ipsilateral single, ≤ 3 cm
N2a	Ipsilateral single, ≤ 3 cm and extranodal extensions *or* Ipsilateral single, > 3 to 6 cm
N2b	Ipsilateral multiple, ≤ 6 cm
N2c	Bilateral, contralateral, ≤ 6 cm
N3a	> 6 cm
N3b	> 3 cm and extranodal extension
M1	Distant metastasis

CARCINOMA OF THE SKIN
OF THE EYELID (ICD-O-3 C44.1)

Rules of Classification

There should be histological confirmation of the disease and division of cases by histological type – for example, basal cell, squamous cell, sebaceous carcinoma. Melanoma of the eyelid is classified with malignant melanoma of skin.

Regional Lymph Nodes

The regional lymph nodes are the preauricular, submandibular and cervical lymph nodes.

TNM Clinical Classification

T – Primary Tumour

T0	No evidence of primary tumour
Tis	Carcinoma in situ
T1	Tumour 10 mm or less in greatest dimension
	T1a Not invading the tarsal plate or eyelid margin (Fig. 346)
	T1b Invades tarsal plate or eyelid margin (Fig. 347)
	T1c Involves full thickness of eyelid (Fig. 348)
T2	Tumour > 10 mm, but 20 mm or less in greatest dimension
	T2a Not invading the tarsal plate or eyelid margin (Fig. 349)
	T2b Invades the tarsal plate or eyelid margin (Fig. 350)
	T2c Involves full thickness of eyelid (Fig. 351)

(a)

T1a   pT1a

(b)

T1a   pT1a

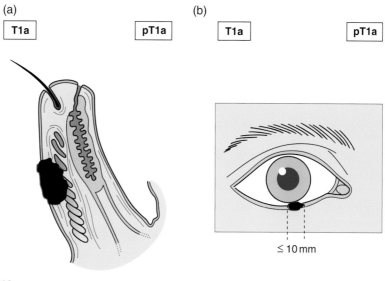

Fig. 346

(a)

T1b   pT1b

(b)

T1b   pT1b

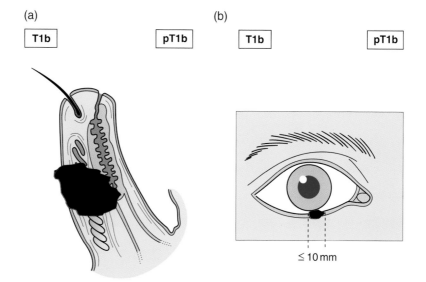

Fig. 347

Skin

(a)

T1c   pT1c

(b)

T1c   pT1c

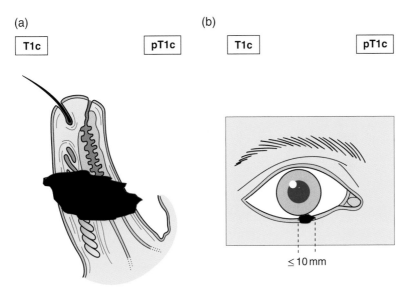

Fig. 348

(a)

T2a   pT2a

(b)

T2a   pT2a

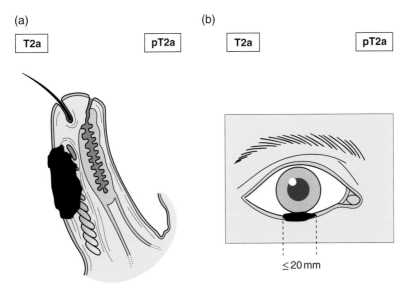

Fig. 349

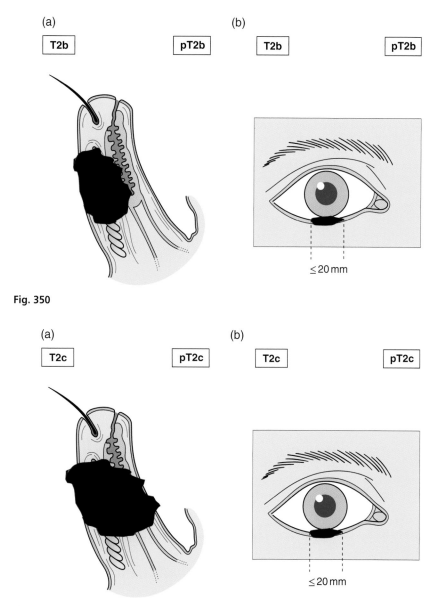

(a)

T2b   pT2b

(b)

T2b   pT2b

≤ 20 mm

Fig. 350

(a)

T2c   pT2c

(b)

T2c   pT2c

≤ 20 mm

Fig. 351

T3   Tumour > 20 mm, but more than 30 mm in greatest dimension
      T3a   Not invading the tarsal plate or eyelid margin (Fig. 352)
      T3b   Invades tarsal plate or eyelid margin (Fig. 353)
      T3c   Involves full thickness of eyelid (Fig. 354)
T4   Any eyelid tumour that invades adjacent ocular, orbital or facial structures
      T4a   Tumour invades ocular or intraorbital structures (Fig. 355a)
      T4b   Tumour invades (or erodes through) the bony walls of the orbit or extends
           to paranasal sinuses or invades the lacrimal sac/nasolacrimal duct or brain
           (Fig. 355b)

(a)   (b)

| T3a | | pT3a | | T3a | | pT3a |

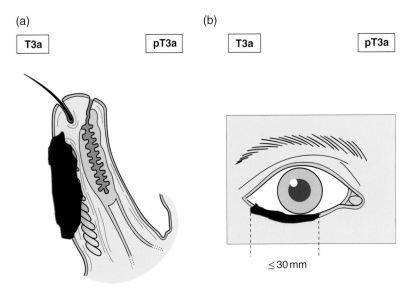

Fig. 352

(a)   (b)

| T3b | | pT3b | | T3b | | pT3b |

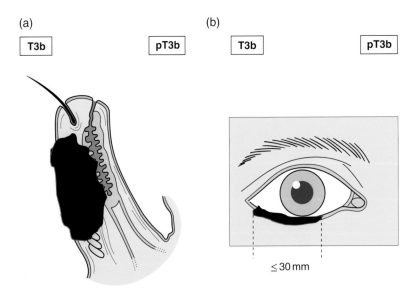

Fig. 353

(a)   (b)

T3c   pT3c   T3c   pT3c

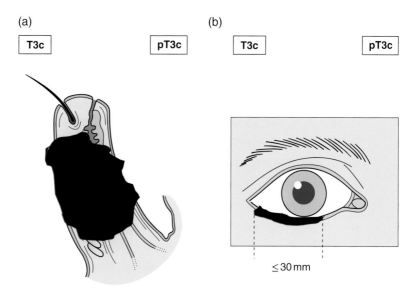

≤ 30 mm

Fig. 354

(a)   (b)
T4a   T4b

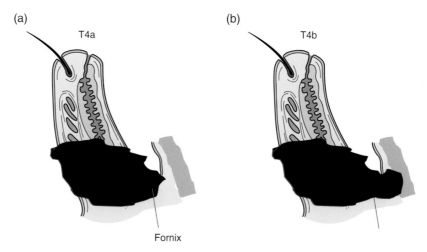

Fornix

Fig. 355

N – Regional Lymph Nodes

NX   Regional lymph nodes cannot be assessed
N0   No evidence of lymph node involvement
N1   Metastasis in a single ipsilateral regional lymph node, 3 cm or less in greatest dimension (Fig. 356a)
N2   Metastasis in a single ipsilateral lymph node more than 3 cm in greatest dimension (Fig. 356b), or in bilateral or contralateral lymph nodes

(a)   (b)

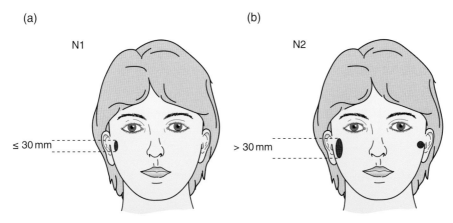

Fig. 356

M – Distant Metastasis

M0   No distant metastasis
M1   Distant metastasis

pTNM Pathological Classification

The pT and pN categories correspond to the T and N categories.

pM1   Distant metastasis microscopically confirmed

Note
pM0 and pMX are not valid categories.

Summary

Eyelid Carcinoma	
T1a	≤ 10 mm, not in tarsal plate or lid margin
T1b	≤ 10 mm, invades tarsal plate or lid margin
T1c	≤ 10 mm, full thickness
T2a	> 10–20 mm, not in tarsal plate or lid margin
T2b	> 10–20 mm, invades tarsal plate or lid margin
T2c	> 10–20 mm, full thickness
T3a	> 20–30 mm, not in tarsal plate or lid margin
T3b	> 20–30 mm, invades tarsal plate or lid margin
T3c	> 20–30 mm, full thickness
T4a	Ocular or intraorbital structures
T4b	Bone, brain, lacrimal sac or nasolacrimal duct
N1	Regional
M1	Distant

MALIGNANT MELANOMA OF SKIN

(ICD-O-3 C44, C51.0, C60.9, C63.2)

Rules for Classification

There should be histological confirmation of the disease.

Regional Lymph Nodes

The regional lymph nodes are those appropriate to the site of the primary tumour. See Regional Lymph Nodes under Skin Tumours.

TNM Clinical Classification

T – Primary Tumour

The extent of the tumour is classified after excision, see pT, page 000.

N – Regional Lymph Nodes

NX   Regional lymph nodes cannot be assessed
N0   No regional lymph node metastasis
N1   Metastasis in one regional lymph node or intralymphatic regional metastasis without nodal metastasis
    N1a   Only microscopic metastasis (clinically occult) (Fig. 357)
    N1b   Macroscopic metastasis (clinically apparent) (Fig. 358)
    N1c   Satellite or in-transit metastasis *without* regional nodal metastasis (Figs. 359, 360)
N2   Metastasis in two or three regional lymph nodes or intralymphatic regional metastasis with regional metastasis
    N2a   Only microscopic nodal metastasis (Fig. 361)
    N2b   Macroscopic nodal metastasis (Fig. 362)
    N2c   Satellite or in-transit metastasis *with only one* regional nodal metastasis (Fig. 363)
N3   Metastasis in four or more regional lymph nodes (Fig. 364), or matted metastatic regional lymph nodes (Fig. 365), or satellite(s) or in-transit metastasis *with* metastasis in regional lymph node(s) (Figs. 366, 367)

Note
Satellites are tumour nests or nodules (macro- or microscopic) within 2 cm of the primary tumour. In-transit metastasis involves skin or subcutaneous tissue more than 2 cm from the primary tumour but not beyond the regional lymph nodes.

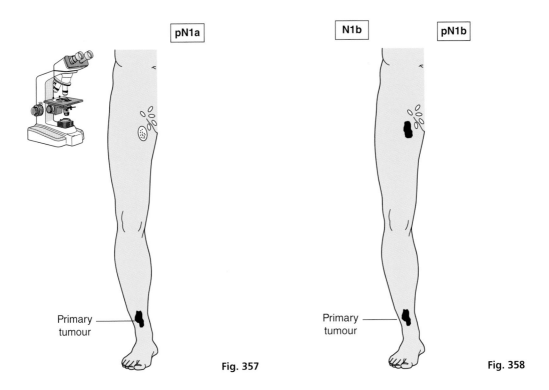

Fig. 357

Fig. 358

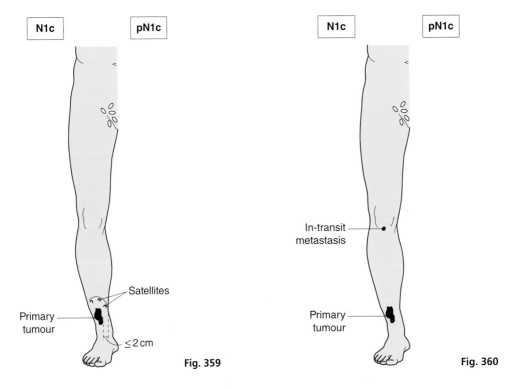

Fig. 359

Fig. 360

Skin

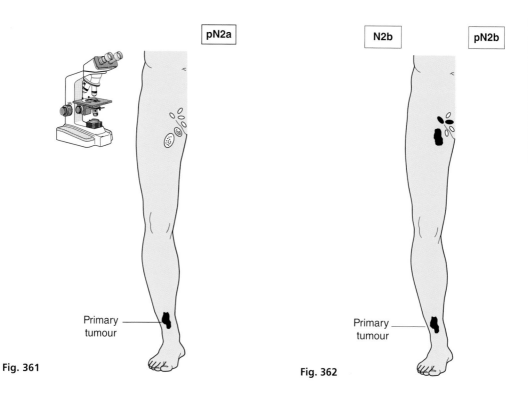

pN2a

Primary
tumour

Fig. 361

N2b   pN2b

Primary
tumour

Fig. 362

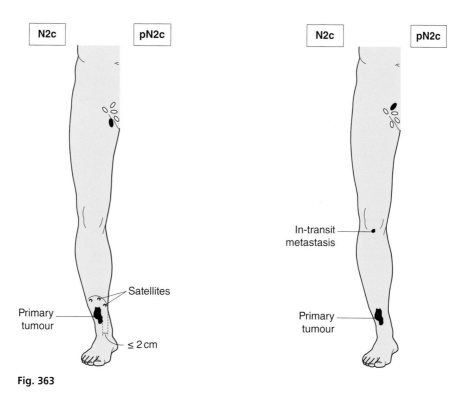

N2c   pN2c

Primary
tumour

Satellites

≤ 2 cm

Fig. 363

N2c   pN2c

In-transit
metastasis

Primary
tumour

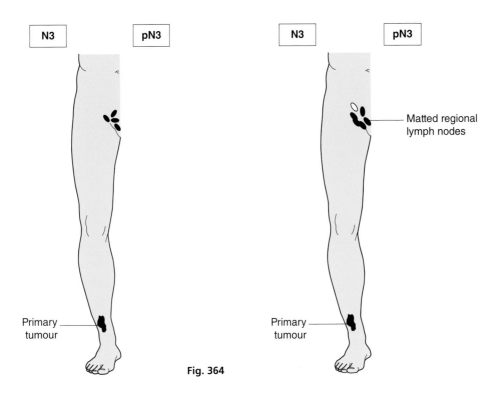

N3   pN3

Matted regional
lymph nodes

Primary
tumour

Fig. 364

N3   pN3

Primary
tumour

Fig. 365

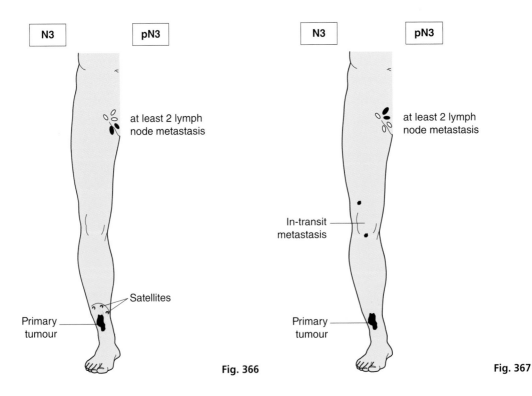

N3   pN3

at least 2 lymph
node metastasis

Satellites

Primary
tumour

Fig. 366

N3   pN3

at least 2 lymph
node metastasis

In-transit
metastasis

Primary
tumour

Fig. 367

M – Distant Metastasis

M0   No distant metastasis
M1   Distant metastasis
    M1a   Skin, subcutaneous tissue or lymph node(s) beyond the regional lymph nodes (Figs. 324, 325, 326, 327)
    M1b   Lung
    M1c   Other sites, or any site with elevated serum lactate dehydrogenase (LDH)

pTNM Pathological Classification

pT – Primary Tumour

The pT classification of malignant melanoma considers the following histological criteria:
1. Tumour thickness (Breslow) according to the largest vertical diameter of the tumour in millimetre (Fig. 368)
2. Absence or presence of ulceration of the primary tumour

(a)

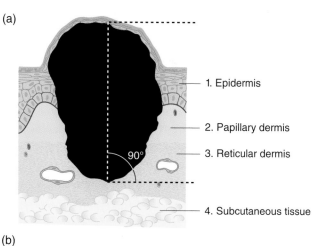

1. Epidermis

2. Papillary dermis

3. Reticular dermis

4. Subcutaneous tissue

(b)

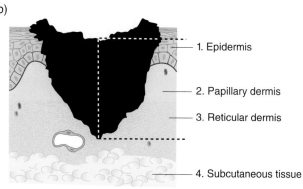

1. Epidermis

2. Papillary dermis

3. Reticular dermis

4. Subcutaneous tissue

Fig. 368

pTX   Primary tumour cannot be assessed*
pT0   No evidence of primary tumour
pTis   Melanoma in situ (Clark level I)

Note
*pTX includes shave biopsies and curettage that do not fully assess the thickness of the primary.

pT1   Tumour 1 mm or less in thickness
      pT1a   Less than 0.8 mm thickness without ulceration (Fig. 369)
      pT1b   Less than 0.8 mm in thickness with ulceration or 0.8 mm or more but
            no more than 1 mm in thickness, with or without ulceration (Fig. 370)
pT2   Tumour more than 1 mm but not more than 2 mm in thickness (Fig. 371)
      pT2a   without ulceration
      pT2b   with ulceration
pT3   Tumour more than 2 mm but not more than 4 mm in thickness (Fig. 372)
      pT3a   without ulceration
      pT3b   with ulceration
pT4   Tumour more than 4 mm in thickness (Fig. 373)
      pT4a   without ulceration
      pT4b   with ulceration

pT1a

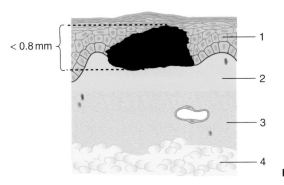

Fig. 369

pT1b

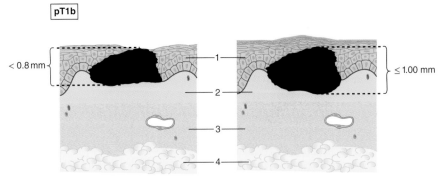

Fig. 370

Skin

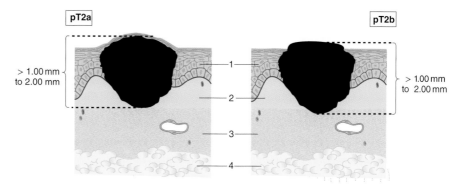

Fig. 371

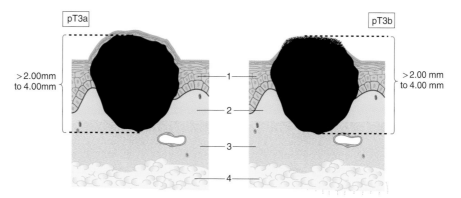

Fig. 372

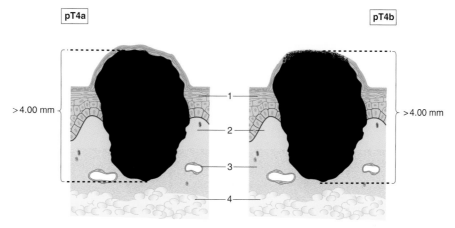

Fig. 373

pN – Regional Lymph Nodes

The pN categories correspond to the N categories. (Figs. 357, 358, 359, 360, 361, 362, 364, 365, 366, 367).

pN0   Histological examination of a regional lymphadenectomy specimen will ordinarily include 6 or more lymph nodes. If the lymph nodes are negative, but the number ordinarily examined is not met, classify as pN0. Classification based solely on sentinel node biopsy without subsequent axillary lymph node dissection is designated (sn) for sentinel node, e.g., pN1(sn). (See Introduction.)

pM – Distant Metastasis

pM1   Distant metastasis microscopically confirmed

Note
pM0 and pMX are not valid categories.

Summary

Skin Malignant Melanoma		
pT1a	< 0.8 mm, no ulceration	
pT1b	< 0.8 mm, ulceration or 0.8–1 mm	
pT2a	> 1–2 mm, no ulceration	
pT2b	> 1–2 mm, ulceration	
pT3a	> 2–4 mm, no ulceration	
pT3b	> 2–4 mm, ulceration	
pT4a	> 4 mm, no ulceration	
pT4b	> 4 mm, ulceration	
N1	1 node or satellite/in-transit without nodes	
	N1a	Microscopic
	N1b	Macroscopic
	N1c	Satellites/in-transit without nodes
N2	2–3 nodes or satellites/in-transit with node	
	N2a	2–3 nodes microscopic
	N2b	2–3 nodes macroscopic
	N2c	Satellite(s) or in-transit with one node
N3	> 4 nodes; matted nodes; satellite(s) or in-transit with >1 nodes	
M1	Distant	
	M1a	Skin, subcutaneous tissues, node(s) beyond regional
	M1b	Lung(s)
	M1c	Other sites, or any sites with elevated LDH

MERKEL CELL CARCINOMA OF SKIN (ICD-O-3 C44.0–9, C63.2)

Rules for Classification

The classification applies only to Merkel cell carcinomas. There should be histological confirmation of the disease.

Regional Lymph Nodes

The regional lymph nodes are those appropriate to the site of the primary tumour. See Regional Lymph Nodes under Skin Tumours.

TNM Clinical Classification

T – Primary Tumour

TX   Primary tumour cannot be assessed
T0   No evidence of primary tumour
Tis   Carcinoma in situ

T1   Tumour 2 cm or less in greatest dimension (Fig. 374)
T2   Tumour more than 2 cm but not more than 5 cm in greatest dimension (Fig. 375)
T3   Tumour more than 5 cm in greatest dimension (Fig. 376)
T4   Tumour invades deep extradermal structures, i.e., cartilage, skeletal muscle, fascia or bone (Fig. 377)

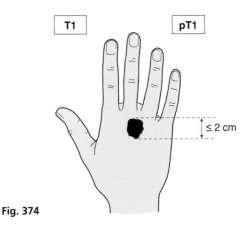

Fig. 374

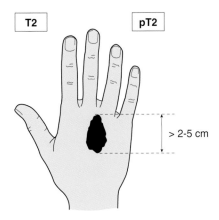

Fig. 375

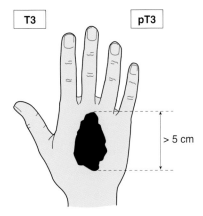

Fig. 376

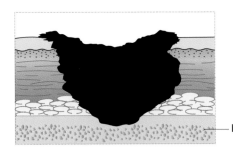

Fig. 377

N – Regional Lymph Nodes

NX   Regional lymph nodes cannot be assessed
N0   No regional lymph node metastasis
N1   Regional lymph node metastasis
N2   In transit metastasis *without* lymph node metastasis
N3   In transit metastasis *with* lymph node metastasis

Note

In-transit metastasis: a tumour distinct from the primary lesion and located between the primary lesion and the draining regional lymph nodes and/or distal to the primary lesion

M – Distant Metastasis

M0   No distant metastasis
M1   Distant metastasis
    M1a   Skin, subcutaneous tissues or non-regional lymph node(s)
    M1b   Lung
    M1c   Other site(s)

pTNM Pathological Classification

The pT category corresponds to the T category.

pNX   Regional lymph nodes cannot be assessed
pN0   No regional lymph node metastasis
pN1   Regional lymph node metastasis
    pN1a(sn)   Microscopic metastasis detected on sentinel node biopsy
    pN1a   Microscopic metastasis detected on node dissection
    pN1b   Macroscopic metastasis (clinically apparent)
pN2   In transit metastasis *without* lymph node metastasis
pN3   In transit metastasis *with* lymph node metastasis

pM1   Distant metastasis microscopically confirmed

Note

pM0 and pMX are not valid categories.

pN0   Histological examination of a regional lymphadenectomy specimen will ordinarily include 6 or more lymph nodes. If the lymph nodes are negative, but the number ordinarily examined is not met, classify as pN0.

Summary

Merkel Cell Carcinoma		
T1	≤ 2 cm	
T2	> 2 to 5 cm	
T3	> 5 cm	
T4	Deep extradermal structures (cartilage, skeletal muscle, fascia, bone)	
N1	Regional	
	pN1a	Microscopic
	pN1b	Macroscopic
N2	In transit metastasis, no lymph node metastasis	
N3	In transit metastasis, lymph node metastasis	
M1	Distant	
	M1a	Skin, subcutaneous tissues or non-regional lymph nodes
	M1b	Lung
	M1c	Other site(s)

BREAST TUMOURS (ICD-O-3 C50)

Rules for Classification

The classification applies only to carcinomas and concerns the male as well as the female breast. There should be histological confirmation of the disease. The anatomical subsite of origin should be recorded but is not considered in classification.

In the case of multiple simultaneous primary tumours in one breast, the tumour with the highest T category should be used for classification. Simultaneous *bilateral* breast cancers should be classified independently to permit division of cases by histological type.

Anatomical Subsites (Fig. 378)

1. Nipple (C50.0)
2. Central portion (C50.1)
3. Upper-inner quadrant (C50.2)
4. Lower-inner quadrant (C50.3)

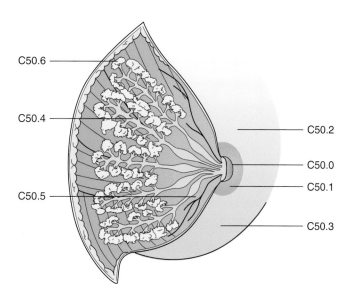

Fig. 378

TNM Atlas: Illustrated Guide to the TNM Classification of Malignant Tumours, Seventh Edition.
Edited by James D. Brierley, Hisao Asamura, Elisabeth Van Eycken, and Brian Rous.
© 2021 by UICC. Published 2021 by John Wiley & Sons Ltd.

5. Upper-outer quadrant (C50.4)
6. Lower-outer quadrant (C50.5)
7. Axillary tail (C50.6)

Regional Lymph Nodes (Fig. 379)

The regional lymph nodes are:
1. *Axillary* (ipsilateral): interpectoral (Rotter) nodes and lymph nodes along the axillary vein and its tributaries, which may be divided into the following levels:
   (i) *Level I* (low-axilla): lymph nodes lateral to the lateral border of pectoralis minor muscle.
   (ii) *Level II* (mid-axilla): lymph nodes between the medial and lateral borders of the pectoralis minor muscle and the interpectoral (Rotter) lymph nodes.
   (iii) *Level III* (apical axilla): apical lymph nodes and those medial to the medial margin of the pectoralis minor muscle, excluding those designated as subclavicular or infraclavicular.
2. *Infraclavicular (subclavicular)* (ipsilateral).
3. *Internal mammary* (ipsilateral): lymph nodes in the intercostal spaces along the edge of the sternum in the endothoracic fascia.
4. *Supraclavicular* (ipsilateral).

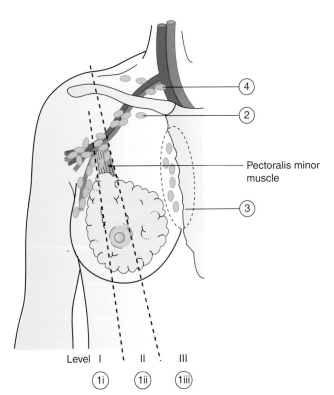

Pectoralis minor muscle

Level I   II   III

Fig. 379

Any other lymph node metastasis is coded as a distant metastasis (M1), including cervical or contralateral internal mammary lymph nodes.

Note
Intramammary lymph nodes are coded as axillary lymph nodes level I.

TNM Clinical Classification

T – Primary Tumour

TX	Primary tumour cannot be assessed
T0	No evidence of primary tumour
Tis	Carcinoma in situ
Tis (DCIS)	Ductal carcinoma in situ
Tis (LCIS)	Lobular carcinoma in situ
Tis (Paget)	Paget disease of the nipple without detectable tumour (Fig. 380)

Note
Tis (Paget) is not associated with invasive carcinoma and/or carcinoma in situ (DCIS and/or LCIS) in the underlying breast parenchyma. Carcinomas in the breast parenchyma associated with Paget disease are categorized based on the size and characteristics of the parenchymal disease, although the presence of Paget disease should still be noted.

T1	Tumour 2 cm or less in greatest dimension
T1mi	Microinvasion 0.1 cm or less in greatest dimension (Fig. 381)

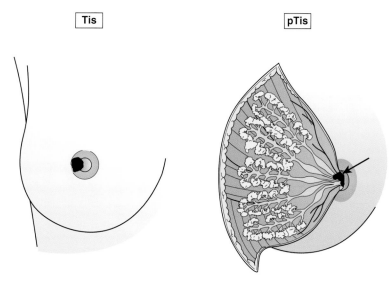

Tis   pTis

Fig. 380

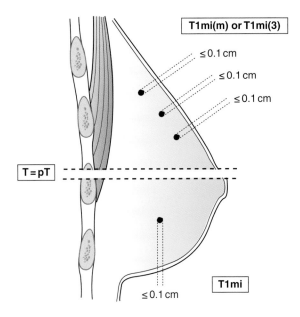

T1mi(m) or T1mi(3)

≤ 0.1 cm

≤ 0.1 cm

≤ 0.1 cm

T = pT

T1mi

≤ 0.1 cm

Fig. 381

Note

Microinvasion is the extension of cancer cells beyond the basement membrane into the adjacent tissues with no focus more than 0.1 cm in greatest dimension. When there are multiple foci of microinvasion, the size of only the largest focus is used to classify the microinvasion. (Do not use the sum of all individual foci.) The presence of multiple foci of microinvasion should be noted, as it is with multiple larger invasive carcinomas.

	T1a	More than 0.1 cm but not more than 0.5 cm in greatest dimension (Fig. 382)
	T1b	More than 0.5 cm but not more than 1 cm in greatest dimension (Fig. 382)
	T1c	More than 1 cm but not more than 2 cm in greatest dimension (Fig. 382)
T2		Tumour more than 2 cm but not more than 5 cm in greatest dimension (Fig. 383)
T3		Tumour more than 5 cm in greatest dimension (Fig. 383)
T4		Tumour of any size with direct extension to chest wall and/or to skin (ulceration or skin nodules).

Note

Invasion of the dermis alone does not qualify as T4. Chest wall includes ribs, intercostal muscles, and serratus anterior muscle but not pectoral muscle.

T4a	Extension to chest wall, not including only pectoralis muscle adherence/invasion (Fig. 384)
T4b	Ulceration and/or ipsilateral satellite skin nodules and/or oedema (including peau d'orange) of the skin which do not meet the criteria for inflammatory carcinoma (Figs. 385, 386)
T4c	Both 4a and 4b, above (Fig. 387)
T4d	Inflammatory carcinoma (Fig. 388)

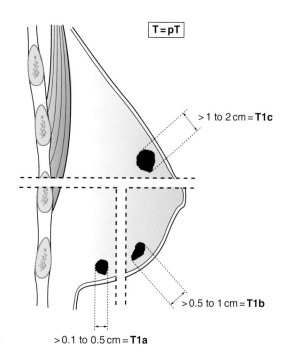

> 1 to 2 cm = **T1c**

> 0.5 to 1 cm = **T1b**

Fig. 382   > 0.1 to 0.5 cm = **T1a**

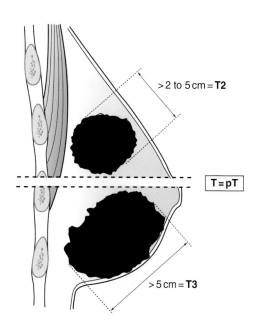

> 2 to 5 cm = **T2**

> 5 cm = **T3**

Fig. 383

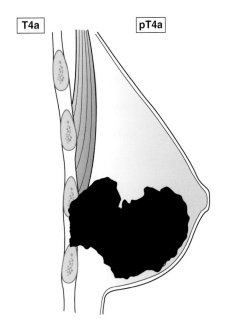

T4a   pT4a

Fig. 384

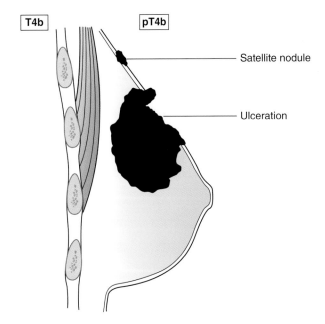

T4b   pT4b

Satellite nodule

Ulceration

Fig. 385

T4b   pT4b

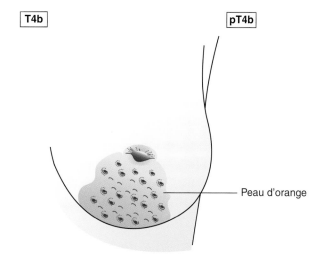

Peau d'orange

Fig. 386

T4c   pT4c

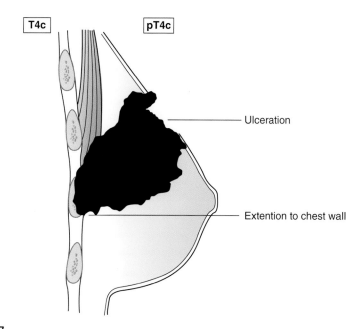

Ulceration

Extention to chest wall

Fig. 387

T4d   pT4d

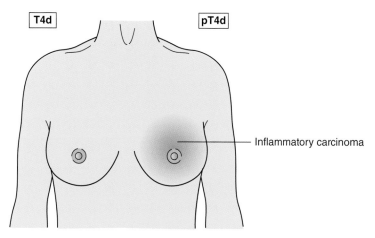

Inflammatory carcinoma

Fig. 388

Note

Inflammatory carcinoma of the breast is characterized by diffuse, brawny induration of the skin with an erysipeloid edge, usually with no underlying mass. If the skin biopsy is negative and there is no localized measurable primary cancer, the T category is pTX when pathologically staging a clinical inflammatory carcinoma (T4d). Dimpling of the skin, nipple retraction, or other skin changes, except those in T4b and T4d, may occur in T1, T2, or T3 without affecting the classification.

N – Regional Lymph Nodes

NX   Regional lymph nodes cannot be assessed (e.g., previously removed)

N0   No regional lymph node metastasis

N1   Metastasis in movable ipsilateral level I, II axillary lymph node(s) (Fig. 389)

N2   Metastasis in ipsilateral level I, II axillary lymph node(s) that are clinically fixed or matted; or in clinically detected* ipsilateral internal mammary lymph node(s) in the *absence* of clinically evident axillary lymph node metastasis

    N2a   Metastasis in axillary lymph node(s) fixed to one another (matted) or to other structures (Fig. 390)

    N2b   Metastasis only in clinically detected* internal mammary lymph node(s) and in the *absence* of clinically evident axillary lymph node metastasis (Fig. 391)

N3   Metastasis in ipsilateral infraclavicular (level III axillary) lymph node(s) with or without level I, II axillary lymph node involvement; or in clinically detected* ipsilateral internal mammary lymph node(s) with clinically evident level I, II axillary lymph node metastasis; or metastasis in ipsilateral supraclavicular lymph node(s) with or without axillary or internal mammary lymph node involvement

    N3a   Metastasis in infraclavicular lymph node(s) (Fig. 392)

N1

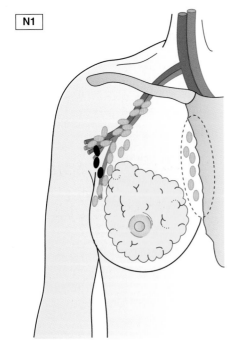

Fig. 389

N2a

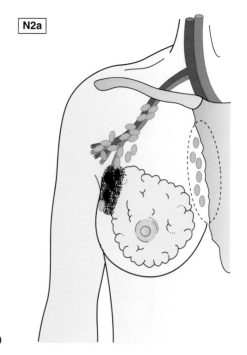

Fig. 390

N2b

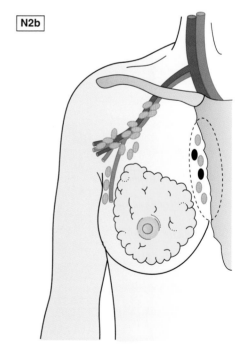

Fig. 391

N3b   Metastasis in internal mammary and axillary lymph nodes (Fig. 393)
N3c   Metastasis in supraclavicular lymph node(s) (Fig. 394)

N3a

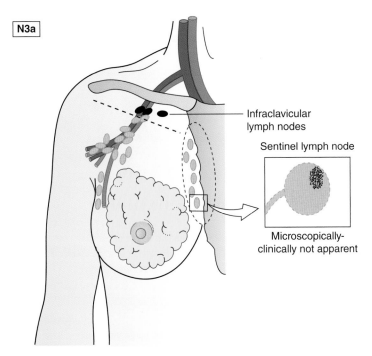

Infraclavicular
lymph nodes

Sentinel lymph node

Microscopically-
clinically not apparent

Fig. 392

N3b

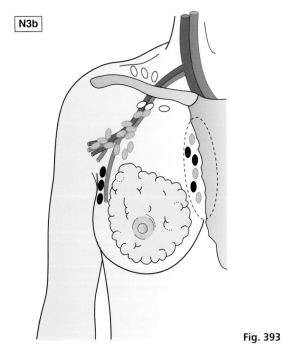

Fig. 393

Breast

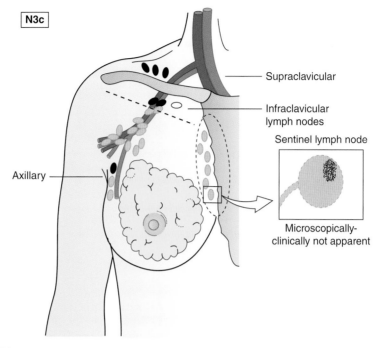

N3c

Supraclavicular

Infraclavicular
lymph nodes

Sentinel lymph node

Axillary

Microscopically-
clinically not apparent

Fig. 394

Note

*Clinically detected is defined as detected by clinical examination or by imaging studies (excluding lymphoscintigraphy) and having characteristics highly suspicious for malignancy or a presumed pathological macrometastasis based on fine needle aspiration biopsy with cytologic examination. Confirmation of clinically detected metastatic disease by fine needle aspiration without excision biopsy is designated with an (f) suffix, e.g. cN3a(f).

Excisional biopsy of a lymph node or biopsy of a sentinel node, in the absence of assignment of a pT, is classified as a clinical N, e.g., cN1. Pathologic classification (pN) is used for excision or sentinel lymph node biopsy only in conjunction with a pathologic T assignment.

M – Distant Metastasis

M0   No distant metastasis
M1   Distant metastasis

pTNM Pathological Classification

pT – Primary Tumour

The pathological classification requires the examination of the primary carcinoma with no gross tumour at the margins of resection. A case can be classified pT if there is only microscopic tumour in a margin.

The pT categories correspond to the T categories.

Note

When classifying pT the tumour size is a measurement of the invasive component. If there is a large in situ component (e.g., 4 cm) and a small invasive component (e.g., 0.5 cm), the tumour is coded pT1a.

pN – Regional Lymph Nodes

The pathological classification requires the resection and examination of at least the low axillary lymph nodes (level I) (see page 2). Such a resection will ordinarily include 6 or more lymph nodes. If the lymph nodes are negative, but the number ordinarily examined is not met, classify as pN0.

pNX   Regional lymph nodes cannot be assessed (e.g., previously removed, or not removed for pathologic study)

pN0   No regional lymph node metastasis*

Note

*Isolated tumour cell clusters (ITC) are single tumour cells or small clusters of cells not more than 0.2 mm in greatest extent that can be detected by routine H and E stains or immunohistochemistry. An additional criterion has been proposed to include a cluster of fewer than 200 cells in a single histological cross section. Nodes containing only ITCs are excluded from the total positive node count for purposes of N classification and should be included in the total number of nodes evaluated (see Introduction).

pN1   Micrometastases; or metastases in 1 to 3 axillary ipsilateral lymph nodes; and/or in internal mammary nodes with metastases detected by sentinel lymph node biopsy but not clinically detected*

pN1mi   Micrometastases (larger than 0.2 mm and/or more than 200 cells, but none larger than 2.0 mm) (Fig. 395)

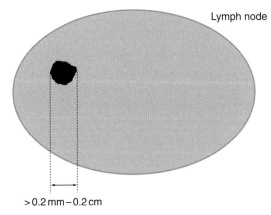

pN1mi

Lymph node

>0.2 mm–0.2 cm

Fig. 395

pN1a   Metastasis in 1–3 axillary lymph node(s), including at least one larger than 2 mm in greatest dimension (Fig. 396)

pN1b   Internal mammary lymph nodes not clinically detected (Fig. 397)

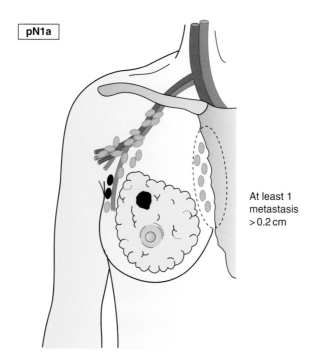

Fig. 396

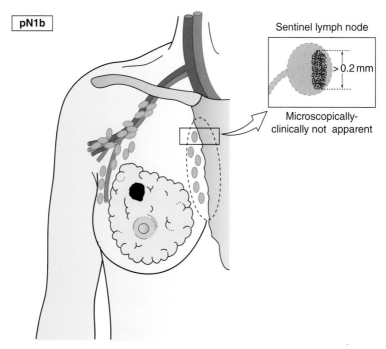

Fig. 397

pN1c   Metastasis in 1–3 axillary lymph nodes and internal mammary lymph nodes not clinically detected (Fig. 398)

pN2   Metastasis in 4–9 ipsilateral axillary lymph nodes, or in clinically detected* ipsilateral internal mammary lymph node(s) in the absence of axillary lymph node metastasis

pN2a   Metastasis in 4–9 axillary lymph nodes, including at least one that is larger than 2 mm (Fig. 399)

pN2b   Metastasis in clinically detected internal mammary lymph node(s), in the *absence* of axillary lymph node metastasis (Fig. 400)

pN3   Metastasis in 10 or more ipsilateral axillary lymph nodes; or in ipsilateral infraclavicular lymph nodes; or in clinically detected ipsilateral internal mammary lymph nodes in the *presence* of one or more positive axillary lymph nodes; or in more than 3 axillary lymph nodes with clinically negative, microscopic metastasis in internal mammary lymph nodes; or in ipsilateral supraclavicular lymph nodes

pN3a   Metastasis in 10 or more axillary lymph nodes (at least one larger than 2 mm) *or* metastasis in infraclavicular lymph nodes/Level III lymph nodes (Figs. 401, 402)

pN3b   Metastasis in clinically detected* internal mammary lymph node(s) in the *presence* of positive axillary lymph node(s) (Fig. 403); or metastasis in more than 3 axillary lymph nodes *and* in internal mammary lymph nodes with microscopic or macroscopic metastasis detected by sentinel lymph node dissection but not clinically detected

pN3c   Metastasis in supraclavicular lymph node(s) (Fig. 404)

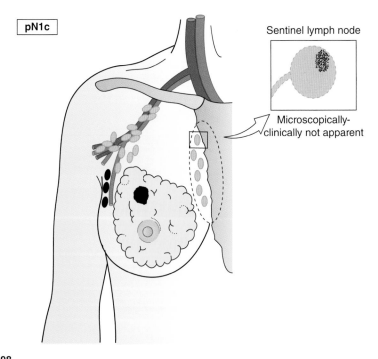

Fig. 398

pN2a

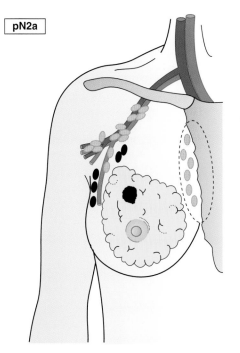

4–9 axillary lymph node metastases, at least 1 metastasis > 2.0 mm

Fig. 399

pN2b

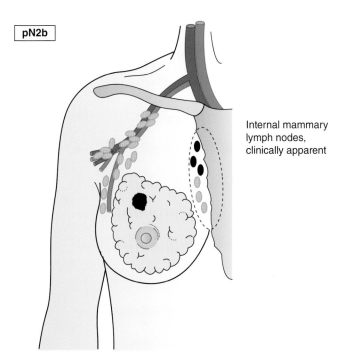

Internal mammary lymph nodes, clinically apparent

Fig. 400

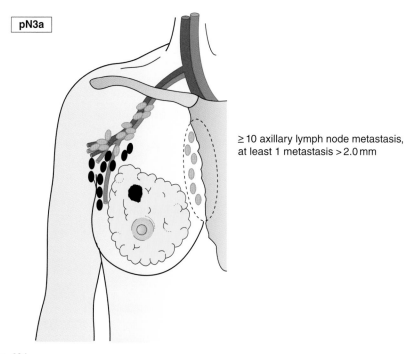

≥ 10 axillary lymph node metastasis,
at least 1 metastasis > 2.0 mm

Fig. 401

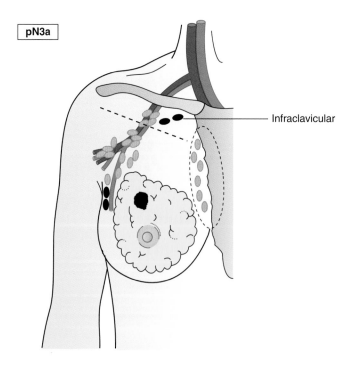

Infraclavicular

Fig. 402

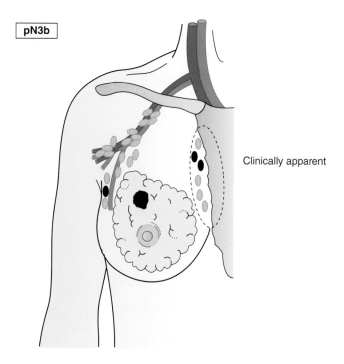

Fig. 403

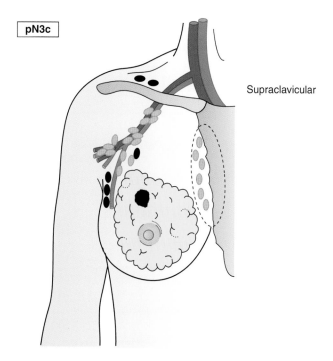

Fig. 404

Post-treatment ypN

- The modifier "sn" is used only if a sentinel node evaluation was performed after treatment. If no subscript is attached, it is assumed the axillary nodal evaluation was by axillary node dissection.
- The X classification will be used (ypNX) if no yp post-treatment SN or axillary dissection was performed
- N categories are the same as those used for pN.

Note

Clinically detected is defined as detected by imaging studies (excluding lymphoscintigraphy) or by clinical examination and having characteristics highly suspicious for malignancy or a presumed pathologic macrometastasis based on fine needle aspiration biopsy with cytologic examination.

Not clinically detected is defined as not detected by imaging studies (excluding lymphoscintigraphy) or not detected by clinical examination.

pM – Distant Metastasis

pM1   Distant metastasis microscopically confirmed

Note

pM0 and pMX are not valid categories.

Summary

Breast			
Tis	in situ		
T1	≤ 2 cm		
T1mi	≤ 0.1 cm		
T1a	> 0.1 to 0.5 cm		
T1b	> 0.5 cm to 1.0 cm		
T1c	> 1.0 to 2.0 cm		
T2	> 2 to 5 cm		
T3	> 5 cm		
T4	Chest wall/skin ulceration		
T4a	Chest wall		
T4b	Skin ulceration, satellite skin nodules		
T4c	Both T4a and T4b		
T4d	Inflammatory carcinoma		
N1 Movable	pN1mi	Micrometastasis > 0.2 mm to 2 mm axillary	
	pN1a	1–3 axillary nodes	
	pN1b	Internal mammary nodes not clinically detected	
	pN1c	1–3 axillary nodes and internal mammary nodes not clinically apparent	
N2a Fixed axillary	pN2a	4–9 axillary nodes	
N2b Internal mammary clinically apparent	pN2b	Internal mammary nodes, clinically detected, without axillary nodes	
N3a Infraclavicular	pN3a	≥ 10 axillary nodes or infraclavicular/Level III lymph nodes	
N3b Internal mammary and axillary	pN3b	Internal mammary nodes, clinically detected, with axillary node(s) or > 3 axillary nodes and internal mammary nodes with microscopic by sentinel node biopsy but not clinically detected	
N3c Supraclavicular	pN3c	Ipsilateral supraclavicular	

GYNAECOLOGICAL TUMOURS

Introductory Notes

The following sites are included:
- Vulva
- Vagina
- Cervix uteri
- Corpus uteri
  - Endometrium
  - Uterine sarcomas
- Ovary, Fallopian tube and primary peritoneal carcinoma
- Gestational trophoblastic tumours

Cervix uteri and corpus uteri were among the first sites to be classified by the TNM system. Originally, carcinoma of the cervix uteri was staged following the rules suggested by the Radiological Sub-Commission of the Cancer Commission of the Health Organization of the "League of Nations." These rules were then adopted, with minor modifications, by the newly formed Fédération Internationale de Gynécologie et d'Obstétrique (FIGO). Finally, UICC brought them into the TNM in order to correspond to the FIGO stages. FIGO, UICC, and AJCC work in close collaboration in the revision process.

TNM Atlas: Illustrated Guide to the TNM Classification of Malignant Tumours, Seventh Edition.
Edited by James D. Brierley, Hisao Asamura, Elisabeth Van Eycken, and Brian Rous.
© 2021 by UICC. Published 2021 by John Wiley & Sons Ltd.

VULVA (ICD-O-3 C51)

The definitions of the T, N, and M categories correspond to the FIGO stages. Both systems are included for comparison.

Rules for Classification

The classification applies only to primary carcinomas of the vulva. There should be histological confirmation of the disease.

A carcinoma of the vulva that has extended to the vagina is classified as carcinoma of the vulva.

The FIGO stages are based on surgical staging. TNM stages are based on clinical and/or pathological classification.

Anatomical Subsites (Fig. 405)

1. Labia majora (C51.0)
2. Labia minora (C51.1)
3. Clitoris (C51.2)

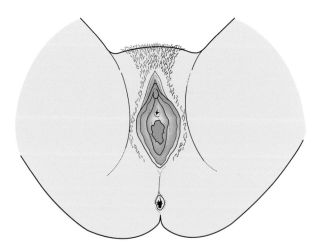

Fig. 405

Regional Lymph Nodes

The regional lymph nodes are the inguinofemoral (groin) nodes.

TNM Clinical Classification

T – Primary Tumour

TX   Primary tumour cannot be assessed

T0   No evidence of primary tumour

Tis   Carcinoma in situ (preinvasive carcinoma), intraepithelial neoplasia grade III (VIN III)

T1   Tumour confined to vulva or vulva and perineum (Fig. 406c)

      T1a   Tumour 2 cm or less in greatest dimension and with stromal invasion no greater than 1.0 mm* (Fig. 406a)

      T1b   Tumour greater than 2 cm or with stromal invasion greater than 1 mm* (Fig. 406b)

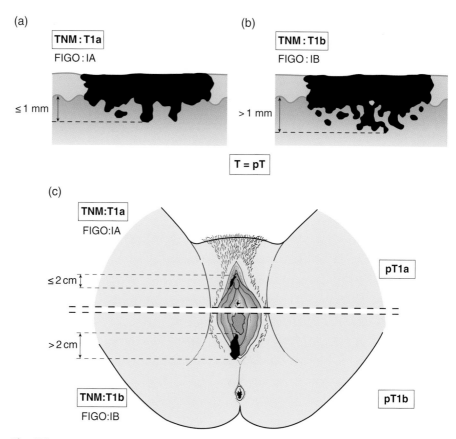

Fig. 406

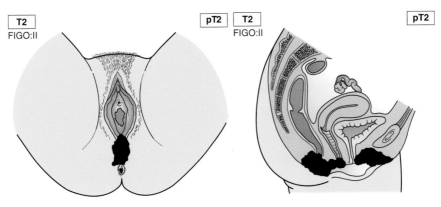

Fig. 407

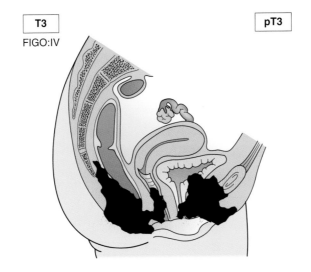

Fig. 408

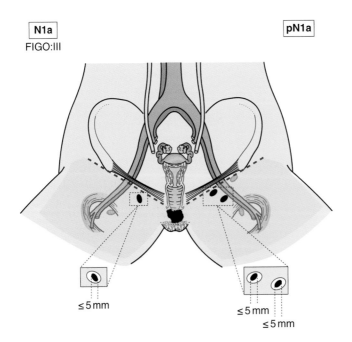

Fig. 409

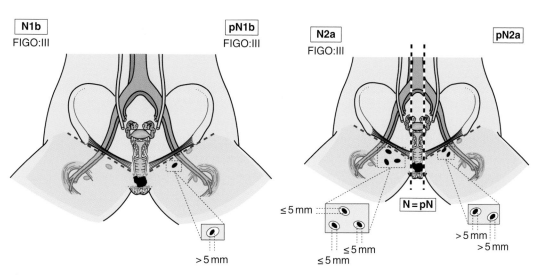

Fig. 410

Fig. 411

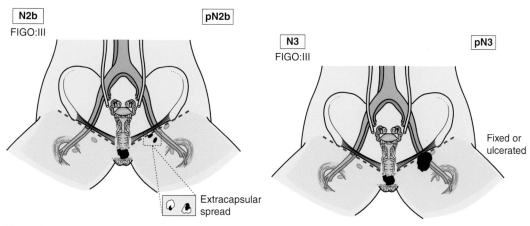

Fig. 412

Fig. 413

T2   Tumour invades any of the following perineal structures: lower third urethra, lower third vagina, anus (Fig. 407)

T3**   Tumour invades any of the following perineal structures: upper 2/3 urethra, upper 2/3 vagina, bladder mucosa, rectal mucosa; or fixed to pelvic bone (Fig. 408)

Notes

*The depth of invasion is defined as the measurement of the tumour from the epithelial–stromal junction of the adjacent most superficial dermal papilla to the deepest point of invasion.

**T3 is not used by FIGO. They label it T4.

N – Regional Lymph Nodes

NX   Regional lymph nodes cannot be assessed

N0   No regional lymph node metastasis

N1   Regional lymph node metastasis with the following features
        N1a   One or two lymph node metastasis less than 5 mm (Fig. 409)
        N1b   One lymph node metastases 5 mm or greater (Fig. 410)
N2   Regional lymph node metastasis with the following features:
        N2a   Three or more lymph node metastases each less than 5 mm (Fig. 411)
        N2b   Two or more lymph node metastases 5 mm or greater (Fig. 412)
        N2c   Lymph node metastasis with extracapsular spread
N3   Fixed or ulcerated regional lymph node metastasis (Fig. 413)

M – Distant Metastasis

M0   No distant metastasis
M1   Distant metastasis (including pelvic lymph node metastasis)

pTN Pathological Classification

The pT and pN categories correspond to the T and N categories.

pM1   Distant metastasis microscopically confirmed

Note
pM0 and pMX are not valid categories.

pN0   Histological examination of an inguinofemoral lymphadenectomy specimen will ordinarily include 6 or more lymph nodes. If the lymph nodes are negative, but the number ordinarily examined is not met, classify as pN0.

Summary

TNM	Vulva	FIGO
T1	Confined to vulva/perineum	I
	T1a ≤ 2 cm with stromal invasion ≤ 1.0 mm	IA
	T1b > 2 cm or stromal invasion > 1.0 mm	IB
T2	Lower urethra/vagina/anus	II
T3	Upper urethra/vagina, bladder rectal/mucosa, bone	IVA
N1a	One or two nodes < 5 mm	IIIA
N1b	One node ≥ 5 mm	IIA
N2a	3 or more nodes < 5 mm	IIIB
N2b	2 or more nodes ≥ 5 mm	IIIB
N2c	Extracapsular spread	IIIC
N3	Fixed or ulcerated	IVA
M1	Distant	IVB

VAGINA (ICD-O-3 C52) (FIG. 414)

The definitions of the T and M categories correspond to the FIGO stages. Both systems are included for comparison.

Rules for Classification

The classification applies to primary carcinomas only. Tumours present in the vagina as secondary growths from either genital or extragenital sites are excluded. A tumour that has extended to the portio and reached the external os (orifice of uterus) is classified as carcinoma of the cervix. A vaginal carcinoma occurring 5 years after successful treatment (complete response) of a carcinoma of the cervix uteri is considered a primary vaginal carcinoma. A tumour involving the vulva is classified as carcinoma of the vulva. There should be histological confirmation of the disease.

The FIGO stages are based on surgical staging. TNM stages are based on clinical and/or pathological classification.

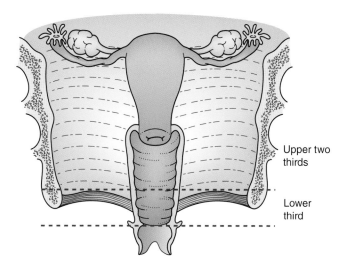

Upper two
thirds

Lower
third

Fig. 414

Regional Lymph Nodes

Upper two-thirds of vagina:

The pelvic nodes including obdurator, internal iliac (hypogastric), external iliac, and pelvic nodes, NOS. (Fig. 415)

Lower third of vagina:

The inguinal and femoral nodes. (Fig. 416)

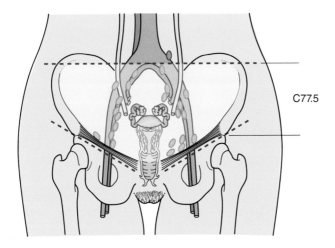

C77.5

Fig. 415

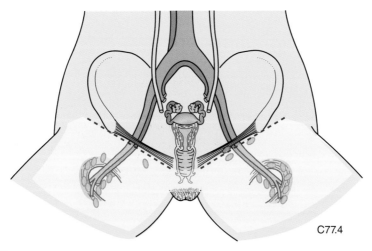

C77.4

Fig. 416

TNM Clinical Classification

T – Primary Tumour

TNM Categories	FIGO Stages	Definition
TX		Primary tumour cannot be assessed
T0		No evidence of primary tumour
Tis	*	Carcinoma in situ (preinvasive carcinoma)
T1	I	Tumour confined to vagina (Fig. 417)
T2	II	Tumour invades paravaginal tissues (paracolpium) (Fig. 418)
T3	III	Tumour extends to pelvic wall (Fig. 419)
T4	IVA	Tumour invades *mucosa* of bladder or rectum, or extends beyond the true pelvis** (Fig. 420)

Note

*FIGO no longer includes Stage 0 (Tis).

**The presence of bullous oedema is not sufficient evidence to classify a tumour as T4.

M1	IVB	Distant metastasis

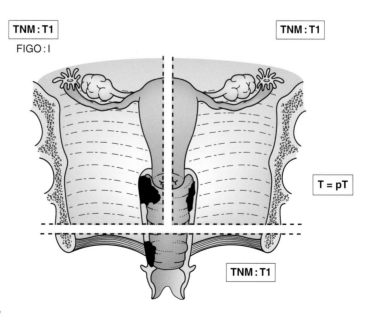

TNM : T1
FIGO : I

TNM : T1

T = pT

TNM : T1

Fig. 417

FIGO : II

pT2

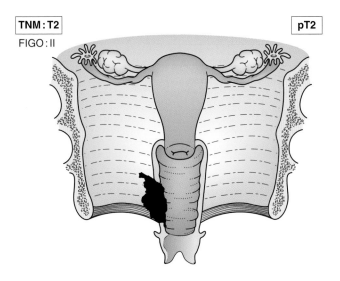

Fig. 418

TNM : T3

FIGO : III

pT3

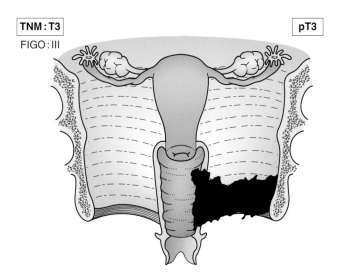

Fig. 419

TNM : T4

FIGO : IV

pT4

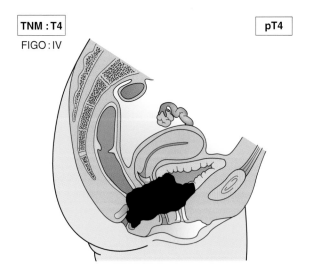

Fig. 420

N – Regional Lymph Nodes

NX   Regional lymph nodes cannot be assessed
N0   No regional lymph node metastasis
N1   Regional lymph node metastasis (Figs. 421, 422, 423)

N1   pN1

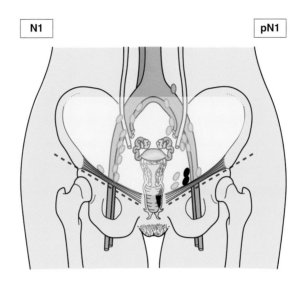

Fig. 421

N1   pN1

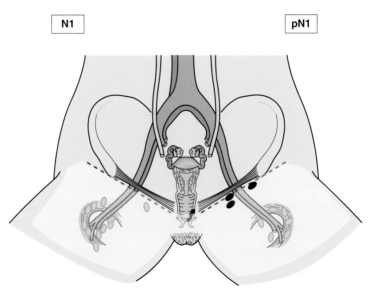

Fig. 422

N1   pN1

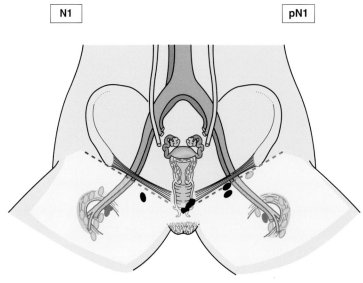

Fig. 423

M – Distant Metastasis

M0   No distant metastasis
M1   Distant metastasis

TNM Pathological Classification

The pT and pN categories correspond to the T and N categories.

pM1   Distant metastasis microscopically confirmed

Note
pM0 and pMX are not valid categories.

pN0 Histological examination of an inguinal lymphadenectomy specimen will ordinarily
include 6 or more lymph nodes; a pelvic lymphadenectomy specimen will ordinarily include 10 or more lymph nodes. If the lymph nodes are negative, but the
number ordinarily examined is not met, classify as pN0.

Gynaecological

Summary

TNM	Vagina	FIGO
T1	Vaginal wall	I
T2	Paravaginal tissue	II
T3	Pelvic wall	III
T4	Mucosa of bladder/rectum, beyond pelvis	IVA
N1	Regional	
M1	Distant metastasis	IVB

CERVIX UTERI (ICD-O-3 C53)

The definitions of the T and M categories correspond to the FIGO stages. Both systems are included for comparison.

Rules for Classification

The classification applies only to carcinomas. There should be histological confirmation of the disease.

FIGO staging of cervical carcinoma was updated in 2018 (ref: DOI: 10.1002/ijgo.12611) and has significant differences to TNM. Please note a new version of TNM staging for cervix is proposed which aligns with the new version of FIGO (see https://www.uicc.org/resources/tnm/publications-resources for details)

Anatomical Subsites (Fig. 424)

1. Endocervix (C53.0)
2. Exocervix (C53.1)

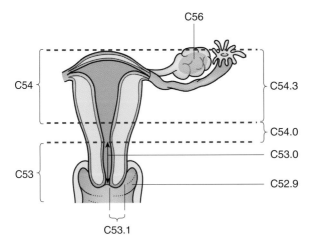

Fig. 424

Regional Lymph Nodes (Fig. 425)

The regional lymph nodes are the paracervical (1), parametrial (2), hypogastric (internal iliac, obturator) (3), common (5) and external iliac (4), presacral (6), lateral sacral nodes (7) and para-aortic nodes (8).

Note

In the 7th edition the para-aortic nodes were considered to be distant metastatic, but to be consistent with advice from FIGO the para-aortic nodes are now classified as regional.

TNM Clinical Classification

T – Primary Tumour

TNM Categories	Definition
TX	Primary tumour cannot be assessed
T0	No evidence of primary tumour
Tis[1]	Carcinoma in situ (preinvasive carcinoma)
T1	Tumour confined to the cervix (extension to corpus should be disregarded)[2]
T1a[3,4]	Invasive carcinoma diagnosed only by microscopy (Fig. 426). Stromal invasion with a maximal depth of 5.0 mm measured from the base of the epithelium and a horizontal spread of 7.0 mm or less[2] (Fig. 427)
T1a1	Measured stromal invasion 3.0 mm or less in depth and 7.0 mm or less in horizontal spread
T1a2	Measured stromal invasion more than 3.0 mm and not more than 5.0 mm with a horizontal spread of 7.0 mm or less (Fig. 428)

Note

[1] FIGO no longer include Stage 0 (Tis)

[2] The depth of invasion should be taken from the base of the epithelium, either surface or glandular, from which it originates. The depth of invasion is defined as the measurement of the tumour from the epithelial–stromal junction of the adjacent most superficial papillae to the deepest point of invasion.

[3] Vascular space involvement, venous or lymphatic, does not affect classification.

[4] FIGO does not consider horizontal extent in definition of IA1 or IA2.

T1b	Clinically visible lesion confined to the cervix (Figs. 429, 431) or microscopic lesion greater than T1a/IA2 (Fig. 430)
T1b1	Clinically visible lesion 4.0 cm or less in greatest dimension[1] (Fig. 429)
T1b2	Clinically visible lesion more than 4.0 cm in greatest dimension[2] (Fig. 431)

Notes

[1] FIGO defines IB1 as Invasive carcinoma $\geq$ 5.0 mm depth of invasion and < 2.0 cm in greatest dimension.

[2] FIGO defines IB2 as Invasive carcinoma $\geq$ 2.0 cm and < 4.0 cm in greatest dimension. FIGO has an additional category of IB3: Invasive carcinoma $\geq$ 4.0 cm in greatest dimension.

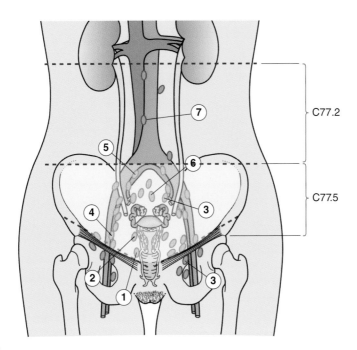

Fig. 425

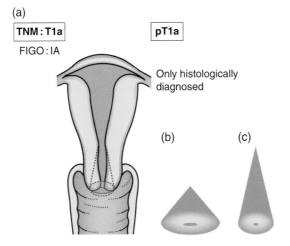

Fig. 426

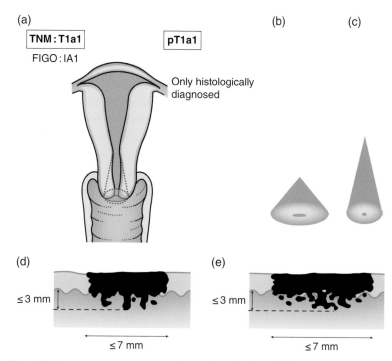

Fig. 427 FIGO does not consider horizontal extent in definition of IA1.

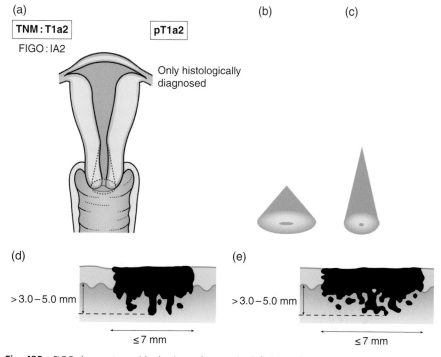

Fig. 428 FIGO does not consider horizontal extent in definition of IA2.

TNM : T1b1   pT1b1

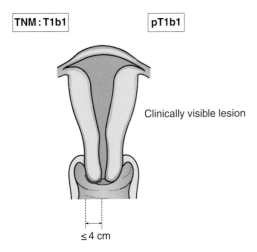

Clinically visible lesion

≤ 4 cm

Fig. 429

(a)

TNM : T1b1   pT1b

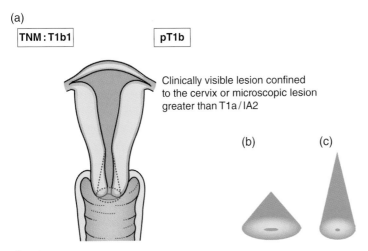

Clinically visible lesion confined
to the cervix or microscopic lesion
greater than T1a / IA2

(b)   (c)

Fig. 430

TNM : T1b2   pT1b2

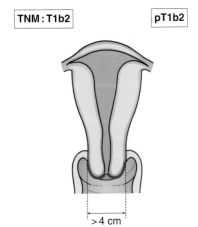

> 4 cm

Fig. 431

Gynaecological

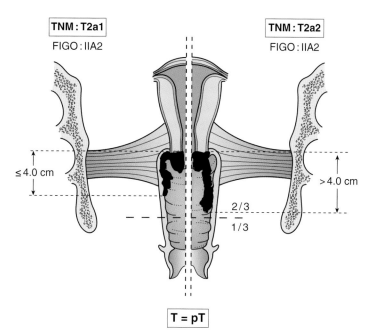

Fig. 432

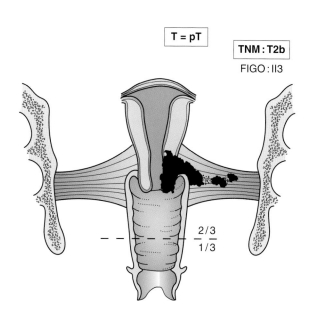

Fig. 433

T2	Tumour invades beyond uterus but not to pelvic wall or to lower third of vagina (Fig. 432)
T2a	Tumour without parametrial invasion
T2a1	Clinically visible lesion 4.0 cm or less in greatest dimension
T2a2	Clinically visible lesion more than 4.0 cm in greatest dimension
T2b	Tumour with parametrial invasion (Fig. 433)
T3	Tumour extends to pelvic wall, involves lower third of vagina, causes hydronephrosis or non-functioning kidney (Fig. 434)
T3a	Tumour involves lower third of vagina
T3b	Tumour extends to pelvic wall, causes hydronephrosis or nonfunctioning kidney
T4	Tumour invades mucosa of the bladder or rectum, or extends beyond true pelvis[1] (Fig. 435)
M1	Distant metastasis

Notes
[1]Bullous oedema is not sufficient to classify a tumour as T4.

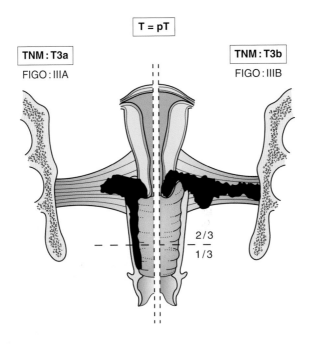

T = pT

TNM : T3a
FIGO : IIIA

TNM : T3b
FIGO : IIIB

2/3
1/3

Fig. 434

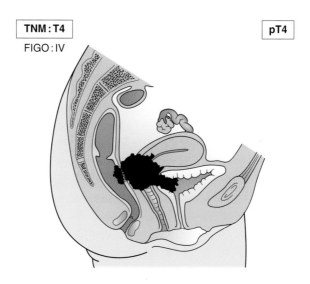

Fig. 435

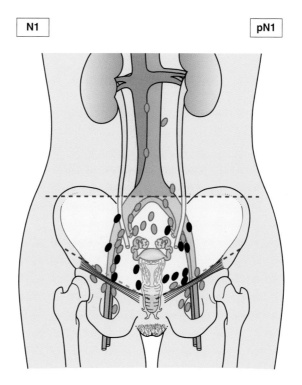

Fig. 436

N – Regional Lymph Nodes

NX   Regional lymph nodes cannot be assessed
N0   No regional lymph node metastasis
N1   Regional lymph node metastasis* (Fig. 436)

Note
FIGO now includes regional lymph nodes in staging of cervical carcinoma. IIIC1 pelvic lymph node metastasis only. IIIC2 para-aortic lymph node metastasis.

M – Distant Metastasis

M0   No distant metastasis
M1   Distant metastasis (includes inguinal lymph nodes and intraperitoneal disease). It excludes metastasis to para-aortic lymph nodes, vagina, pelvic serosa, and adnexa

pTNM Pathological Classification

The pT and pN categories correspond to the T and N categories.

pM1   Distant metastasis microscopically confirmed

Note
pM0 and pMX are not valid categories.

pN0   Histological examination of a pelvic lymphadenectomy specimen will ordinarily include 10 or more lymph nodes. If the lymph nodes are negative, but the number ordinarily examined is not met, classify as pN0.

Gynaecological

Summary

TNM	Cervix Uteri
Tis	Carcinoma in situ
T1	Confined to uterus
T1a	Diagnosed only by microscope
T1a1	Depth $\leq$ 3 mm, horizontal spread $\leq$ 7 mm
T1a2	Depth > 3–5 mm, horizontal spread $\leq$ 7 mm
T1b	Clinically visible or microscopic lesion greater than T1a2
T1b1	$\leq$ 4 cm
T1b2	> 4 cm
T2	Beyond uterus, but not pelvic wall or lower third vagina
T2a	No parametrium
T2a1	$\leq$ 4 cm
T2a2	> 4 cm
T2b	Parametrium
T3	Lower third of vagina, pelvic wall, hydronephrosis, non-functioning kidney
T3a	Lower third of vagina
T3b	Pelvic wall, hydronephrosis, non-functioning kidney
T4	Mucosa bladder/rectum, beyond pelvis
N1	Regional
M1	Distant metastasis

UTERUS ENDOMETRIUM (ICD-O-3 C54.0, 1, 3, 8, 9, C55)

The definitions of the T, N, and M categories correspond to the FIGO stages. Both systems are included for comparison.

Rules for Classification

The classification applies to endometrial carcinomas and carcinosarcomas (malignant mixed mesodermal tumours). There should be histological verification with subdivision by histological type and grading of the carcinomas. The diagnosis should be based on examination of specimens taken by endometrial biopsy.

The FIGO stages are based on surgical staging. TNM stages are based on clinical and/or pathological classification.

Anatomical Subsites (Fig. 424)

1. Isthmus uteri (C54.0)
2. Fundus uteri (C54.3)
3. Endometrium (C54.1)

Regional Lymph Nodes (Fig. 425)

The regional lymph nodes are the pelvic (hypogastric [obturator, internal iliac] (3), common (5) and external (4) iliac, parametrial (2), and sacral (6)) and the para-aortic nodes (7).

TNM Clinical Classification

T – Primary Tumour

TNM Categories	FIGO Stages	Definition
TX		Primary tumour cannot be assessed
T0		No evidence of primary tumour
T1	I*	Tumour confined to the corpus uteri[1] (Fig. 437)
T1a	IA*	Tumour limited to the endometrium or invading less than half of myometrium
T1b	IB	Tumour invades one half or more of myometrium
T2	II	Tumour invades cervical stroma, but does not extend beyond the uterus[2] (Fig. 438)
T3	III	Local and/or regional spread as specified below
T3a	IIIA	Tumour invades the serosa of the corpus uteri or adnexae (direct extension or metastasis) (Fig. 439)
T3b	IIIB	Vaginal or parametrial involvement (direct extension or metastasis) (Fig. 439)
N1	IIIC	Metastasis to pelvic or para-aortic lymph nodes (Fig. 441)
	IIIC1	Metastasis to pelvic lymph nodes
	IIIC2	Metastasis to para-aortic lymph nodes with or without metastasis to pelvic lymph nodes
T4	IVA	Tumour invades bladder/bowel mucosa[3] (Fig. 440)
M1	IVB	Distant metastasis

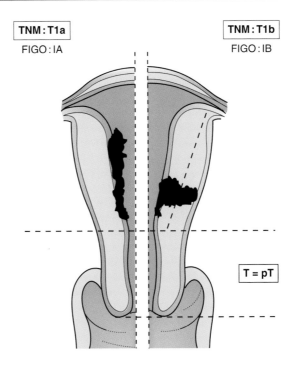

TNM: T1a
FIGO: IA

TNM: T1b
FIGO: IB

T = pT

Fig. 437

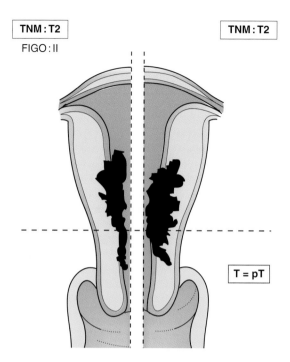

TNM : T2
FIGO : II

TNM : T2

T = pT

Fig. 438

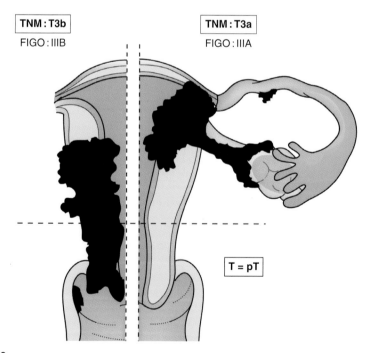

TNM : T3b
FIGO : IIIB

TNM : T3a
FIGO : IIIA

T = pT

Fig. 439

TNM : T4
FIGO : IV

pT4

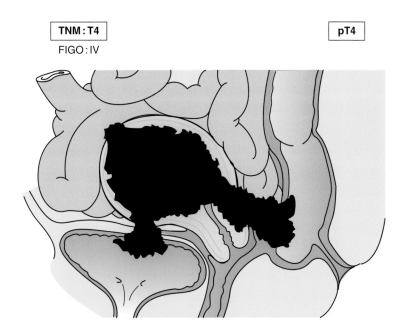

Fig. 440

N2

pN2

Para-aortic nodes

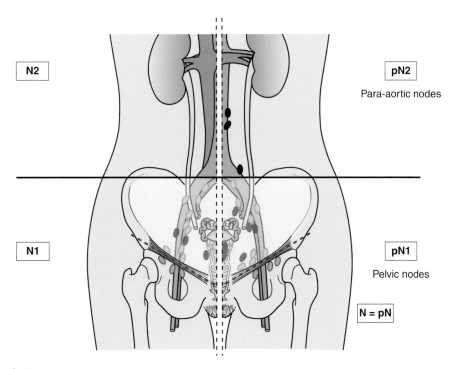

N1

pN1

Pelvic nodes

N = pN

Fig. 441

Notes

[1] Endocervical glandular involvement only should now be considered as stage I.

[2] Positive cytology has to be reported separately without changing the stage.

[3] The presence of bullous oedema is not sufficient evidence to classify as T4.

N – Regional Lymph Nodes

NX   Regional lymph nodes cannot be assessed
N0   No regional lymph node metastasis
N1   Pelvic lymph node metastasis
N2   Para-aortic lymph node metastasis

M – Distant Metastasis

M0   No distant metastasis
M1   Distant metastasis (excluding metastasis to vagina, pelvic serosa, or adnexa, including metastasis to inguinal lymph nodes, intra-abdominal lymph nodes other than para-aortic or pelvic nodes)

pTNM Pathological Classification

The pT and pN categories correspond to the T and N categories.

pM1   Distant metastasis microscopically confirmed

Note
pM0 and pMX are not valid categories.

pN0   Histological examination of a pelvic lymphadenectomy specimen will ordinarily include 6 or more lymph nodes. If the lymph nodes are negative, but the number ordinarily examined is not met, classify as pN0.

Summary

TNM	Endometrium	FIGO
T1	Confined to the uterus (including endocervical gland)	I
T1a	Limited to endometrium, less than half of the myometrium	IA
T1b	Half or more of myometrium	IB
T2	Invades cervix, but not beyond uterus	II
T3	Local and/or regional invasion as described below	III
T3a	Serosa and/or adnexae (direct extension or metastasis)	IIIA
T3b	Vagina, parametrium (direct extension or metastasis)	IIIB
N1/N2	Pelvic and/or para-aortic nodes	IIIC
N1	Pelvic nodes	IIIC1
N2	Para-aortic nodes	IIIC2
T4	Mucosa of bladder/bowel	IVA
M1	Distant metastasis	IVB

UTERUS – UTERINE SARCOMAS

(LEIOMYOSARCOMA, ENDOMETRIAL STROMAL SARCOMA,

ADENOSARCOMA) (ICD-O-3 C53, 54, 55)

The definitions of the T, N, and M categories correspond to the FIGO stages. Both systems are included for comparison.

Rules for Classification

The classification applies to sarcomas except for carcinosarcoma, which is classified as carcinoma of the endometrium. There should be histological confirmation and division of cases by histologic type.

The FIGO stages are based on surgical staging. TNM stages are based on clinical and/ or pathological classification.

Anatomical Subsites (Fig. 424)

1. Cervix uteri (C53)
2. Isthmus uteri (C54.0)
3. Fundus uteri (C54.3)

Histological Types of Tumours

Leiomyosarcoma	ICD-O-3 M 8890/3
Endometrial stromal sarcoma	ICD-O-3 M 8930/3
Endometrial stromal sarcoma, low grade	ICD-O-3 M 8931/3
Adenosarcoma	ICD-O-3 M 8933/3

Regional Lymph Nodes (Fig. 425)

The regional lymph nodes are the pelvic (hypogastric [obturator, internal iliac] (3), common (5) and external (4) iliac, parametrial (2), and sacral (6)) and the para-aortic nodes (7).

Leiomyosarcoma, Endometrial stromal sarcoma

TNM Clinical Classification

T – Primary Tumour

TNM Categories	FIGO Stages	Definition
T1	I	Tumour limited to the uterus
T1a	IA	Tumour 5 cm or less in greatest dimension (Fig. 442)
T1b	IB	Tumour more than 5 cm in greatest dimension (Fig. 443)
T2	II	Tumour extends beyond the uterus, within the pelvis (Fig. 444)
T2a	IIA	Tumour involves adnexa (Fig. 444)
T2b	IIB	Tumour involves other pelvic tissues (Fig. 445)
T3	III	Tumour infiltrates abdominal tissues
T3a	IIIA	One site (Fig. 446)
T3b	IIIB	More than one site (Fig. 447)
N1	IIIC	Metastasis to regional lymph nodes
T4	IVA	Tumour invades bladder or rectum (Fig. 448)
M1	IVB	Distant metastasis

Note

Simultaneous tumours of the uterine corpus and ovary/pelvis in association with ovarian/pelvic endometriosis should be classified as independent primary tumours.

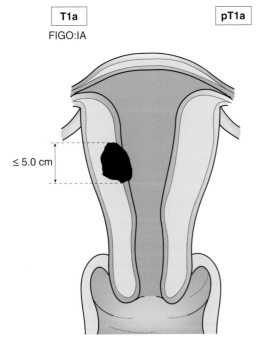

| T1a | pT1a |

FIGO:IA

≤ 5.0 cm

Fig. 442

T1b
FIGO:IB

pT1b

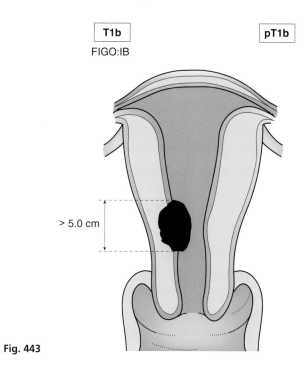

> 5.0 cm

Fig. 443

T2a
FIGO:IA

pT2a

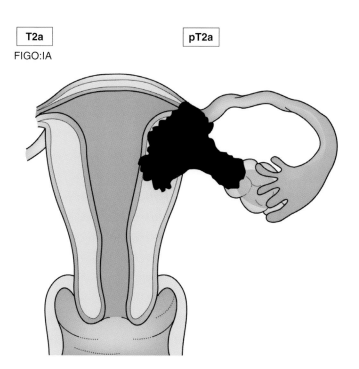

Fig. 444

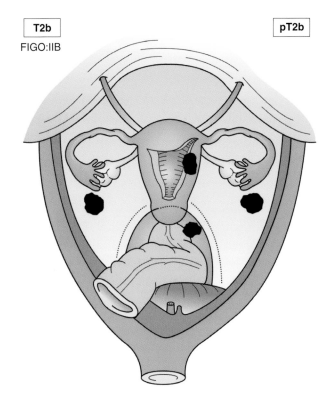

T2b
FIGO:IIB

pT2b

Fig. 445

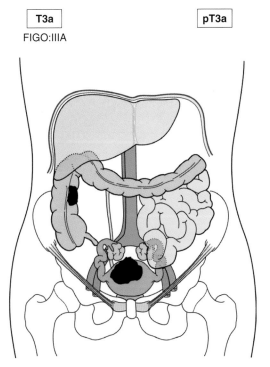

T3a
FIGO:IIIA

pT3a

Fig. 446

T3b

pT3b

FIGO:IIIB

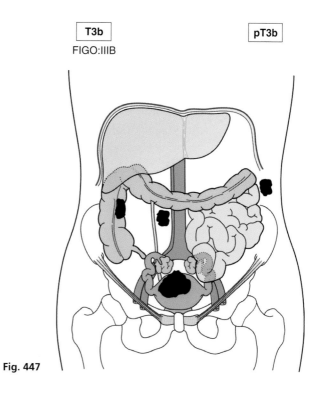

Fig. 447

TNM:T4

pT4

FIGO:IVA

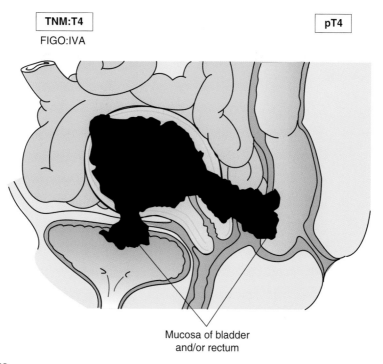

Mucosa of bladder
and/or rectum

Fig. 448

Adenosarcoma

TNM Clinical Classification

T – Primary Tumour

TNM Categories	FIGO Stage	Definition
T1	I	Tumour limited to the uterus
T1a	IA	Tumour limited to the endometrium/endocervix (Fig. 449)
T1b	IB	Tumour invades to less than half of the myometrium (Fig. 450)
T1c	IC	Tumour invades more than half of the myometrium (Fig. 451)
T2	II	Tumour extends beyond the uterus, within the pelvis
T2a	IIA	Tumour involves adnexa (Fig. 444)
T2b	IIB	Tumour involves other pelvic tissues (Fig. 445)
T3	III	Tumour involves abdominal tissues
T3a	IIIA	One site (Fig. 446)
T3b	IIIB	More than one site (Fig. 447)
N1	IIIC	Metastasis to regional lymph nodes
T4	IVA	Tumour invades bladder or rectum (Fig. 448)
M1	IVB	Distant metastasis

Note

Simultaneous tumours of the uterine corpus and ovary/pelvis in association with ovarian/pelvic endometriosis should be classified as independent primary tumours.

T1a
FIGO:IA

pT1a

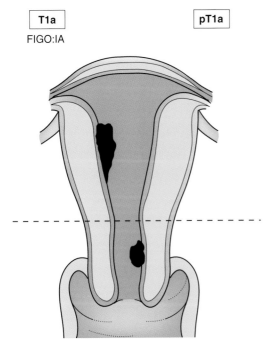

Fig. 449

T1b   pT1b

FIGO:IB

1/2

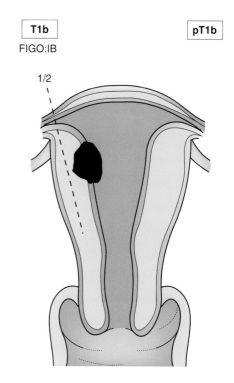

Fig. 450

T1c   pT1c

FIGO:IC

1/2

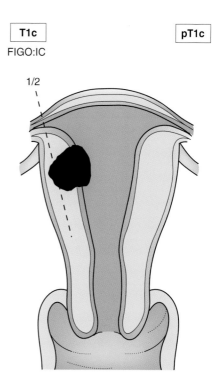

Fig. 451

N – Regional Lymph Nodes

NX   Regional lymph nodes cannot be assessed
N0   No regional lymph node metastasis
N1   Regional lymph node metastasis

M – Distant Metastasis

M0   No distant metastasis
M1   Distant metastasis (excluding adnexa, pelvic and abdominal tissues)

pTNM Pathological Classification

The pT and pN categories correspond to the T and N categories.

pM1   Distant metastasis microscopically confirmed

Note
pM0 and pMX are not valid categories.

Summary

TNM	Uterine Sarcomas	FIGO
T1	Uterus	I
T2	Within pelvis	II
T3	Abdominal tissues	III
T4	Bladder/rectal mucosa	IVA
N1	Regional	
M1	Distant	IVB

OVARIAN, FALLOPIAN TUBE AND PRIMARY PERITONEAL CARCINOMA

(ICD-O-3 C56, C57, C48.1, C48.2)

The definitions of the T, N, and M categories correspond to the FIGO stages. Both systems are included for comparison.

Rules for Classification

The classification applies to malignant ovarian neoplasms of both epithelial and stromal origin, including those of borderline malignancy or of low malignant potential corresponding to "common epithelial tumours" of the earlier terminology. The classification also applies to carcinoma of the Fallopian tubes and to carcinomas of the peritoneum (Müllerian origin). There should be histological confirmation of the disease and division of cases by histological type.

The FIGO stages are based on surgical staging. TNM stages are based on clinical and/or pathological classification.

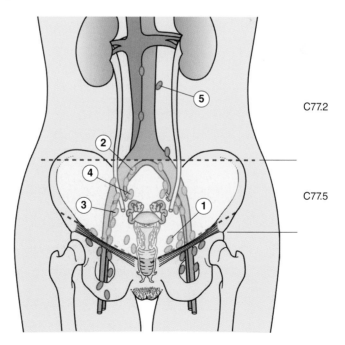

C77.2

C77.5

Fig. 452

Regional Lymph Nodes (Fig. 452)

The regional lymph nodes are the hypogastric (obturator and internal iliac) (1), common iliac (2), external iliac (3), lateral sacral (4) and para-aortic (5).

TNM Clinical Classification

T – Primary Tumour

TNM categories			FIGO stage	Definition
TX				Primary tumour cannot be assessed
T0				No evidence of primary tumour
T1			I	Tumour confined to the ovaries (one or both) or fallopian tube(s)
	T1a		IA	Tumour limited to one ovary (capsule intact) or fallopian tube; no tumour on ovarian or fallopian tube surface, no malignant cells in ascites or peritoneal washings (Fig. 453)
	T1b		IB	Tumour limited to both ovaries or fallopian tubes (Fig. 454)
	T1c		IC	Tumour limited to one or both ovaries or fallopian tubes with any of the following:
		T1c1		Surgical spill
		T1c2		Capsule ruptured before surgery or tumour on ovarian or fallopian tube surface
		T1c3		Malignant cells in ascites or peritoneal washings (Fig. 455)
T2			II	Tumour involves one or both ovaries or fallopian tubes with pelvic extension (below the pelvic brim) or primary peritoneal cancer
	T2a		IIA	Extension and/or implants on uterus and/or fallopian tube(s) and or ovary(ies) (Fig. 456)
	T2b		IIB	Extension to other pelvic tissues, including bowel within the pelvis (Fig. 457)
T3 and/or N1			III[a]	Tumour involves one or both ovaries or fallopian tubes or primary peritoneal carcinoma with cytologically or histologically confirmed spread to the peritoneum outside the pelvis and/or metastasis to the retroperitoneal lymph nodes
N1				Retroperitoneal lymph node metastasis only
	N1a		IIIA1i	Lymph node metastasis not more than 10 mm in greatest dimension (Fig. 458)
	N1b		IIIA1ii	Lymph node metastasis more than 10 mm in greatest dimension (Fig. 458)
T3a any N			IIIA2	Microscopic extrapelvic (above the pelvic brim) peritoneal involvement with or without retroperitoneal lymph node, including bowel involvement (Fig. 459)

T3b any N	IIIB	Macroscopic peritoneal metastasis beyond pelvic brim 2 cm, or less in greatest dimension, including bowel involvement outside the pelvis with or without retroperitoneal nodes (Fig. 459)
T3c any N	IIIC	Peritoneal metastasis beyond pelvic brim more than 2 cm in greatest dimension and/or retroperitoneal lymph node metastasis (includes extension of tumour to capsule of liver and spleen without parenchymal involvement of either organ) (Fig. 459, 460)
M1	IV	Distant metastasis (excludes peritoneal metastasis)
M1a	IVA	Pleural effusion with positive cytology
M1b[b]	IVB	Parenchymal metastasis and metastasis to extra abdominal organs (including inguinal lymph nodes and lymph nodes outside the abdominal cavity) (Fig. 460)

Notes

[a]Liver capsule metastasis is T3/stage III.
[b]Liver parenchymal metastasis M1/stage IV.

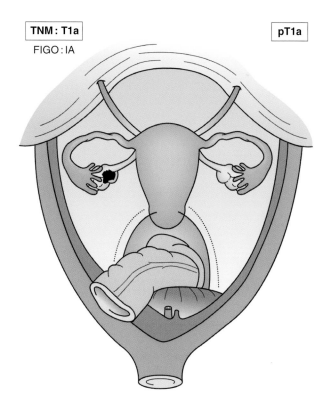

TNM: T1a

FIGO: IA

pT1a

Fig. 453

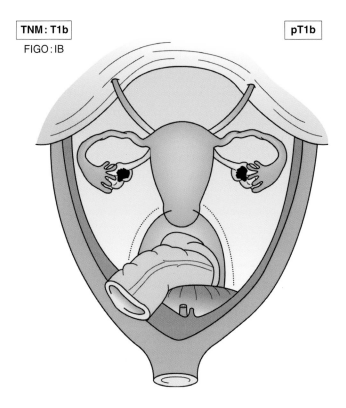

TNM: T1b
FIGO: IB

pT1b

Fig. 454

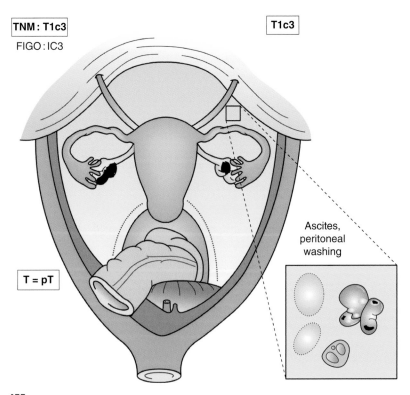

TNM: T1c3
FIGO: IC3

T1c3

Ascites,
peritoneal
washing

T = pT

Fig. 455

TNM : T2a
FIGO : IIA

pT2a

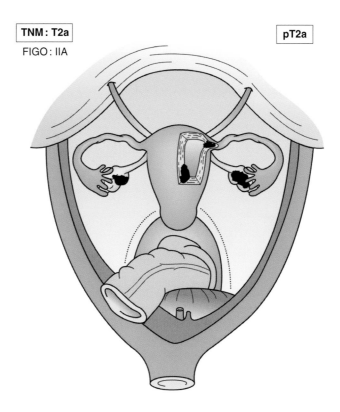

Fig. 456

TNM : T2b
FIGO : IIB

pT2b

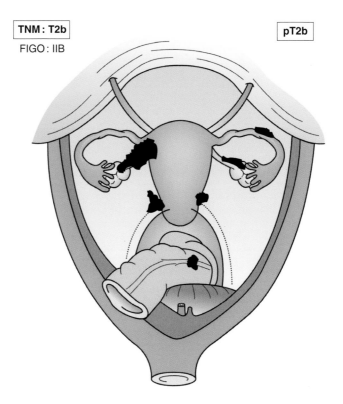

Fig. 457

N1   pN1

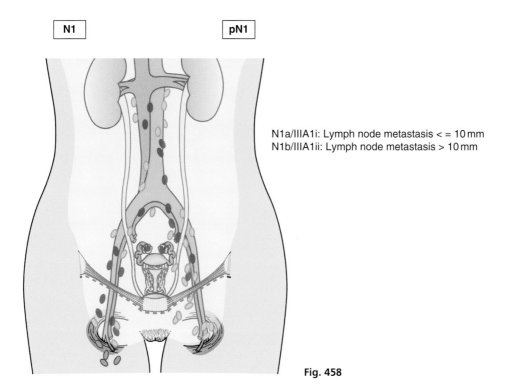

N1a/IIIA1i: Lymph node metastasis < = 10 mm
N1b/IIIA1ii: Lymph node metastasis > 10 mm

Fig. 458

TNM:T3   T3
FIGO:IIIA2–IIIC

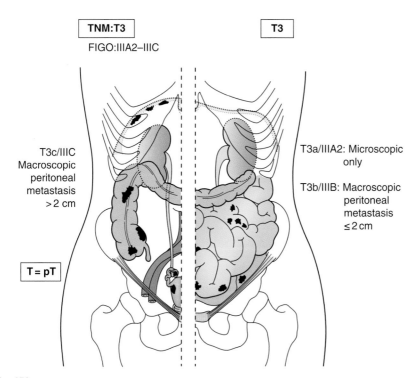

T3c/IIIC
Macroscopic
peritoneal
metastasis
> 2 cm

T3a/IIIA2: Microscopic
only

T3b/IIIB: Macroscopic
peritoneal
metastasis
≤ 2 cm

T = pT

Fig. 459

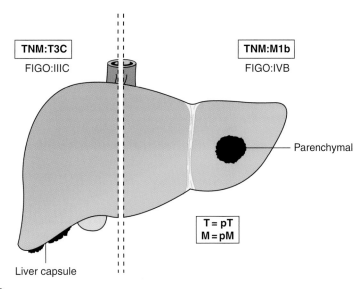

Fig. 460

N – Regional Lymph Nodes

NX   Regional lymph nodes cannot be assessed
N0   No regional lymph node metastasis
N1   Regional lymph node metastasis (Fig. 458)
N1   IIIA1   Retroperitoneal lymph node metastasis only
N1a IIIA1i   Lymph node metastasis no more than 10 mm in greatest dimension
N1b IIIA1ii Lymph node metastasis more than 10 mm in greatest dimension

M – Distant Metastasis

M0   No distant metastasis
M1   Distant metastasis
M1a   Pleural effusion with positive cytology
M1b   Parenchymal metastasis and metastasis to extra-abdominal organs (including inguinal lymph nodes and lymph nodes outside the abdominal cavity) (Fig. 460)

pTNM Pathological Classification

The pT and pN categories correspond to the T and N categories.

pM1   Distant metastasis microscopically confirmed
pM1a   Pleural effusion with positive cytology
pM1b   Parenchymal metastasis and metastasis to extra-abdominal organs (including inguinal lymph nodes and lymph nodes outside the abdominal cavity)

Note

pM0 and pMX are not valid categories.

pN0   Histological examination of a pelvic lymphadenectomy specimen will ordinarily include 6 or more lymph nodes. If the lymph nodes are negative, but the number ordinarily examined is not met, classify as pN0.

Summary

TNM	Ovary	FIGO
T1	Limited to the ovaries or fallopian tubes	I
T1a	One ovary or fallopian tube, capsule/serosal surface intact	IA
T1b	Both ovaries or fallopian tubes, capsule/serosal surface intact	IB
T1c	Capsule ruptured, tumour on ovarian or tubal surface, malignant cells in ascites or peritoneal washings	IC
T1c1	Surgical spill	IC1
T1c2	Capsule rupture or tumour on surface	IC2
T1c3	Positives peritoneal washings	IC3
T2	Pelvic extension	II
T2a	Uterus, tube(s) ovaries	IIA
T2b	Other pelvic tissues	IIB
N1	Regional lymph node metastasis	
N1a	Lymph node metastasis ≤ 10 mm	IIIA1i
N1b	Lymph node metastasis < 10 mm	IIIA1ii
T3	Peritoneal metastasis beyond pelvis	III
T3a	Microscopic peritoneal metastasis	IIIA2
T3b	Macroscopic peritoneal metastasis ≤ 2.0 cm	IIIB
T3c	Peritoneal metastasis > 2.0 cm	IIIC
M1	Distant metastasis (excludes peritoneal metastasis)	IV
M1a	Pleural effusion with positive cytology	IVA
M1b	Parenchymal metastasis and metastasis to extra-abdominal organs	IVB

GESTATIONAL TROPHOBLASTIC TUMOURS (ICD-O-3 C58)

The following classification for gestational trophoblastic tumours is based on that of FIGO adopted in 1992 and updated in 2001 (Ngan HYS, Bender H, Benedet JL, Jones H, Montrucolli GC, Pecorelli S (FIGO Committee on Gynecologic Oncology). Gestational trophoblastic neoplasia. *Int J Gynecol Obstet* 2002; 77:285–287).

The definitions of T and M categories correspond the FIGO stages. Both systems are included for comparison. In contrast to other sites, an N (regional lymph node) classification does not apply to these tumours. A prognostic scoring index, which is based on factors other than the anatomic extent of the disease, is used to assign cases to high risk and low risk categories, and these categories are used in stage grouping.

Rules for Classification

The classification applies to choriocarcinoma (9100/3), invasive hydatidiform mole (9100/1), and placental site trophoblastic tumour (9104/1). Placental site tumours should be reported separately. Histological confirmation is not required if the human chorionic gonadotropin (ßhCG) level is abnormally elevated. History of prior chemotherapy for this disease should be noted.

TNM Clinical Classification

T – Primary Tumour/M – Distant Metastasis

TNM Categories	FIGO Stages*	Definition
TX		Primary tumour cannot be assessed
T0		No evidence of primary tumour
T1	I	Tumour confined to the uterus (Fig. 461)
T2	II	Tumour extends to other genital structures: vagina, ovary, broad ligament, fallopian tube(s), by direct extension or metastasis (Fig. 462)
M1a	III	Metastasis to lung(s)
M1b	IV	Other distant metastasis

Note
*Stage I to IV are subdivided into A and B according to the prognostic score.

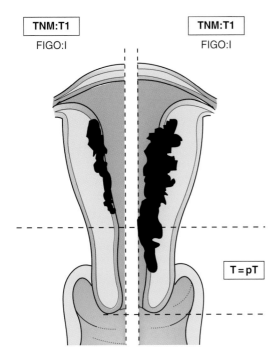

TNM:T1
FIGO:I

TNM:T1
FIGO:I

T = pT

Fig. 461

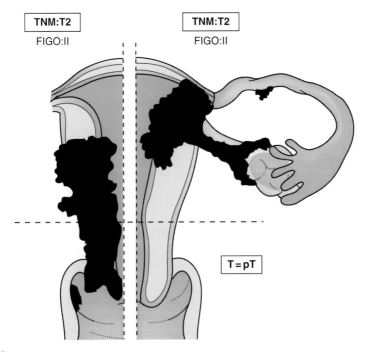

TNM:T2
FIGO:II

TNM:T2
FIGO:II

T = pT

Fig. 462

M – Distant Metastasis

M0	No distant metastasis
M1	Distant metastasis
M1a	Metastasis to lung(s)
M1b	Other distant metastasis

Note

Genital metastasis (vagina, ovary, broad ligament, fallopian tube) is classified T2. Any involvement of non-genital structures, whether by direct invasion or metastasis, is described using the M classification.

pTM Pathological Classification

The pT and pM categories correspond to the T and M categories.

Prognostic Score

Prognostic Factor	0	1	2	4
Age	< 40	≥ 40		
Antecedent pregnancy	H. mole	Abortion	Term pregnancy	
Months from index pregnancy	< 4	4–6	7–12	> 12
Pretreatment serum ßhCG (IU/ml)	$< 10^3$	$10^3-< 10^4$	$10^4-< 10^5$	$\geq 10^5$
Largest tumour size including uterus	< 3 cm	3–5 cm	> 5 cm	
Sites of metastasis	Lung	Spleen, kidney	Gastrointestinal tract	Liver, brain
Number of metastasis		1–4	5–8	> 8
Previous failed chemotherapy			Single drug	Two or more drugs

Summary

TNM and risk	Gestational Trophoblastic Tumours	FIGO
T1	Confined to uterus	I
T2	Other genital structures	II
M1a	Metastasis to lung(s)	III
M1b	Other distant metastasis	IV
Low risk	Prognostic score 6 or less	IA – IVA
High risk	Prognostic score 7 or more	IB – IVB

UROLOGICAL TUMOURS

Introductory Notes

The following sites are included:
- Penis
- Prostate
- Testis
- Kidney
- Renal pelvis and ureter
- Urinary bladder
- Urethra

TNM Atlas: Illustrated Guide to the TNM Classification of Malignant Tumours, Seventh Edition.
Edited by James D. Brierley, Hisao Asamura, Elisabeth Van Eycken, and Brian Rous.
© 2021 by UICC. Published 2021 by John Wiley & Sons Ltd.

PENIS (ICD-O-3 C60)

Rules for Classification

The classification applies only to carcinomas. There should be histological confirmation of the disease.

Anatomical Subsites (Fig. 463)

1. Prepuce (C60.0)
2. Glans penis (C60.1)
3. Body of penis (C60.2)

Regional Lymph Nodes

The regional lymph nodes are the superficial and deep inguinal and the pelvic nodes.

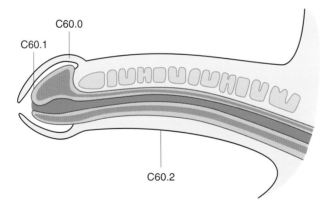

Fig. 463

TNM Clinical Classification

T – Primary Tumour

TX	Primary tumour cannot be assessed
T0	No evidence of primary tumour
Tis	Carcinoma in situ (penile intraepithelial neoplasia – PeIN)
Ta	Noninvasive localized squamous cell carcinoma[1] (Fig. 464)
T1	Tumour invades subepithelial connective tissue[2] (Figs. 465, 466)

      T1a   Tumour invades subepithelial connective tissue without lymphovascular invasion or perineural invasion and is not poorly differentiated

      T1b   Tumour invades subepithelial connective tissue with lymphovascular invasion or perineural invasion or is poorly differentiated

T2	Tumour invades corpus spongiosum with or without invasion of the urethra (Figs. 467, 468)
T3	Tumour invades corpus cavernosum with or without invasion of the urethra (Figs. 467, 468)
T4	Tumour invades other adjacent structures (Figs. 469, 470)

Notes

[1]Including verrucous carcinoma.

[2]Glans: Tumour invades lamina propria.

Foreskin: Tumour invades dermis, lamina propria or dartos fascia.

Shaft: Tumour invades connective tissue between epidermis and corpora and regardless of location.

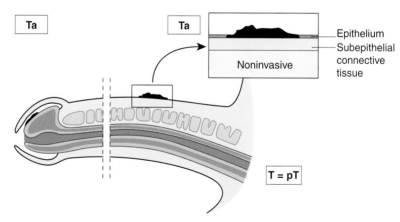

Fig. 464

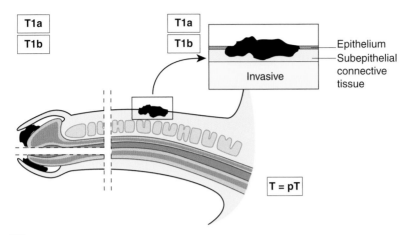

Fig. 465

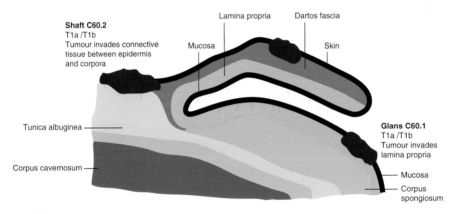

Fig. 466

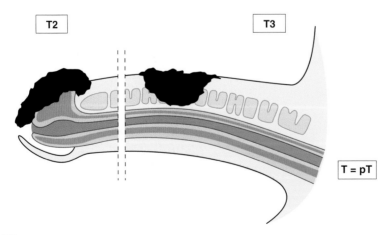

Fig. 467

T2   T3

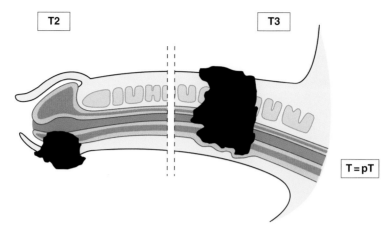

T = pT

Fig. 468

T4   pT4

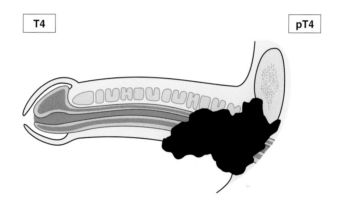

Fig. 469

T4   pT4

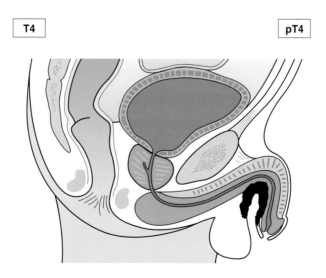

Fig. 470

N – Regional Lymph Nodes

NX   Regional lymph nodes cannot be assessed
N0   No palpable or visibly enlarged inguinal lymph nodes
N1   Palpable mobile unilateral inguinal lymph node (Fig. 471)

N1

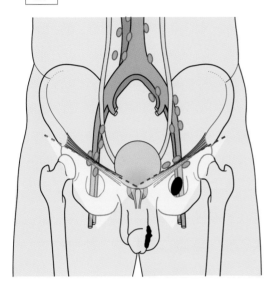

Fig. 471

N2   Palpable mobile multiple (Fig. 472) or bilateral inguinal lymph nodes (Fig. 473)

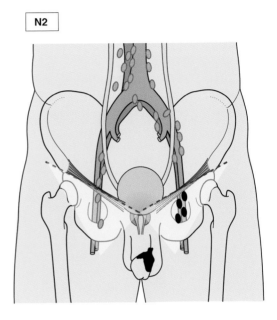

Fig. 472

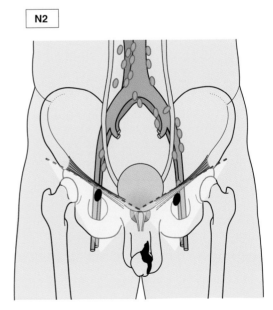

Fig. 473

N3   Fixed inguinal nodal mass (Fig. 474) or pelvic lymphadenopathy unilateral (Fig. 475) or bilateral (Fig. 476)

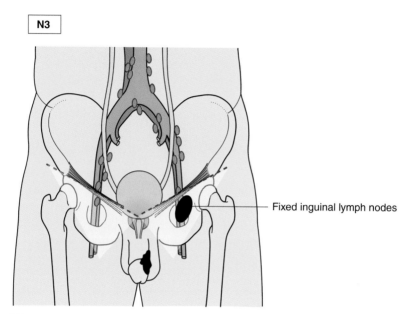

Fixed inguinal lymph nodes

Fig. 474

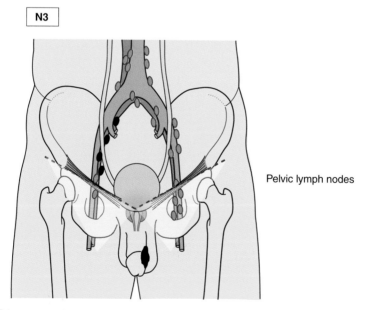

Pelvic lymph nodes

Fig. 475

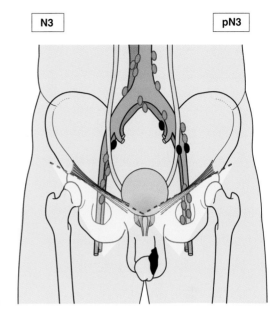

Fig. 476

M – Distant Metastasis

M0   No distant metastasis
M1   Distant metastasis

pTNM Pathological Classification

The pT categories correspond to the T categories. The pN categories are based upon biopsy, or surgical excision.

pNX   Regional lymph nodes cannot be assessed
pN0   No regional lymph node metastasis
pN1   Metastasis in one or two inguinal lymph nodes
pN2   Metastasis in more than two unilateral or bilateral inguinal lymph nodes
pN3   Metastasis in pelvic lymph node(s), unilateral or bilateral or extranodal extension of regional lymph node metastasis
pM1   Distant metastasis microscopically confirmed

Note
pM0 and pMX are not valid categories.

Summary

Penis			
Ta	Noninvasive localized squamous cell carcinoma		
T1	Subepithelial connective tissue		
T1a	Without lymphovascular invasion or perineural invasion, not G3–4		
T1b	With lymphovascular invasion or perineural invasion or G3–4		
T2	Corpus spongiosum with or without invasion of the urethra		
T3	Corpus cavernosum with or without invasion of the urethra		
T4	Other adjacent structures		
N1	Palpable mobile single inguinal	pN1	One or two inguinal
N2	Palpable mobile multiple/bilateral inguinal	pN2	More than 2 unilateral/bilateral inguinal
N3	Fixed inguinal or pelvic	pN3	Pelvic or extranodal
M1	Distant		

PROSTATE (ICD-O-3 C61) (FIG. 477, SEE ALSO FIG. 524)

Rules for Classification

The classification applies only to adenocarcinomas. Transitional cell carcinoma of the prostate is classified as a urethral tumour (see Urethra). There should be histological confirmation of the disease.

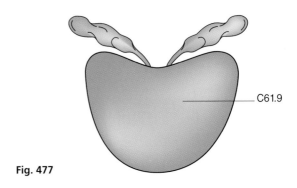

C61.9

Fig. 477

Regional Lymph Nodes (Fig. 478)

The regional lymph nodes are the nodes of the true pelvis, which essentially are the pelvic nodes below the bifurcation of the common iliac arteries. Laterality does not affect the N classification.

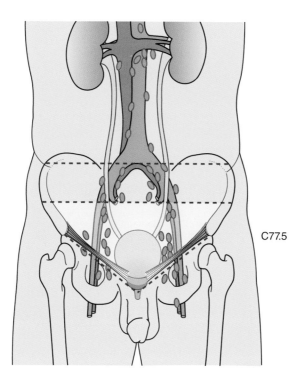

C77.5

Fig. 478

TNM Clinical Classification

T – Primary Tumour

TX   Primary tumour cannot be assessed

T0   No evidence of primary tumour

T1   Clinically inapparent tumour that is not palpable (Fig. 479)
      T1a   Tumour incidental histological finding in 5% or less of tissue resected
      T1b   Tumour incidental histological finding in more than 5% of tissue resected
      T1c   Tumour identified by needle biopsy (e.g., because of elevated PSA)

T2   Tumour that is palpable and confined within prostate[1]
      T2a   Tumour involves one half of one lobe or less (Fig. 480)
      T2b   Tumour involves more than half of one lobe, but not both lobes (Fig. 480)

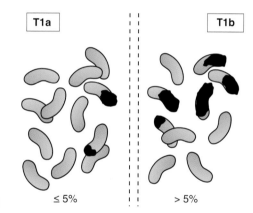

Fig. 479

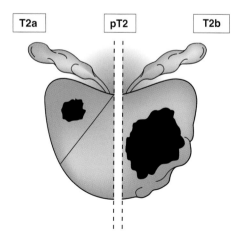

Fig. 480

T2c Tumour involves both lobes (Fig. 481)
T3 Tumour extends through the prostatic capsule[2]
    T3a Extraprostatic extension (unilateral or bilateral) including microscopic bladder neck involvement (Figs. 482, 483)

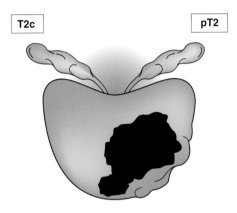

Fig. 481

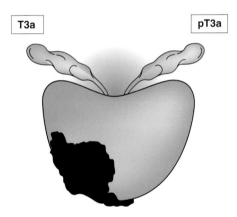

Fig. 482

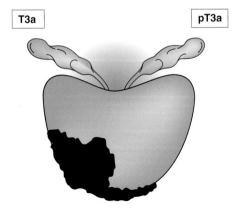

Fig. 483

T3b   Tumour invades seminal vesicle(s) (Fig. 484)

T4   Tumour is fixed or invades adjacent structures other than seminal vesicles: bladder neck, external sphincter, rectum, levator muscles, and/or pelvic wall (Figs. 485, 486)

Notes

[1] Tumour found in one or both lobes by needle biopsy, but not palpable, is classified as T1c.

[2] Invasion into the prostatic apex or into (but not beyond) the prostatic capsule is not classified as T3, but as T2.

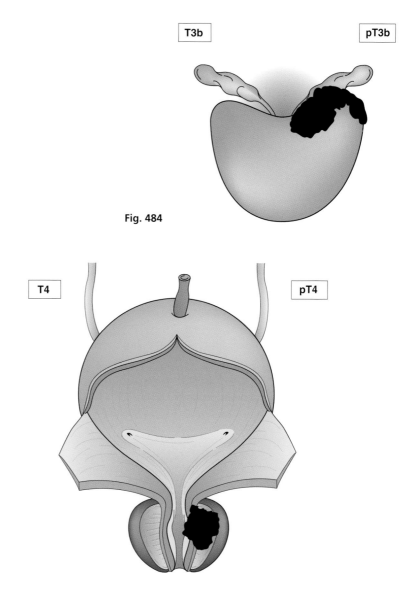

T3b   pT3b

Fig. 484

T4   pT4

Fig. 485

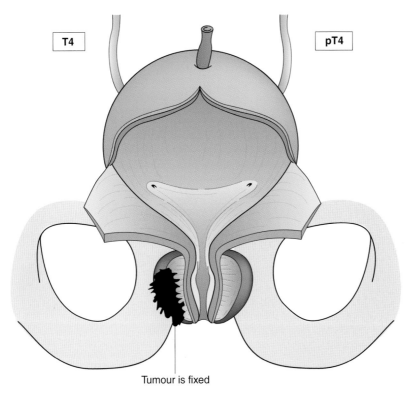

Tumour is fixed

Fig. 486

N – Regional Lymph Nodes

NX   Regional lymph nodes cannot be assessed
N0   No regional lymph node metastasis
N1   Regional lymph node metastasis (Figs. 487, 488)

Note
Metastasis *no* larger than 0.2 cm can be designated pN1mi.

N1   pN1

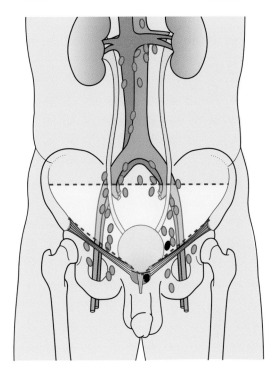

Fig. 487

N1   pN1

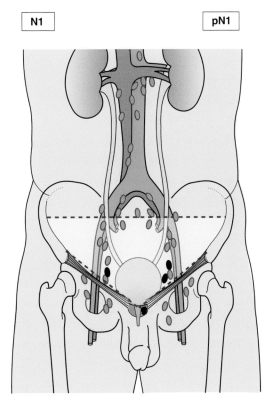

Fig. 488

M – Distant Metastasis*

M0   No distant metastasis
M1   Distant metastasis
        M1a   Non-regional lymph node(s)
        M1b   Bone(s)
        M1c   Other site(s)

Note

*When more than one site of metastasis is present, the most advanced category is used. pM1c is the most advanced category.

pTNM Pathological Classification

The pT and pN categories correspond to the T and N categories.

However, there is no pT1 category because there is insufficient tissue to assess the highest pT category. There are no subcategories of pT2.

pM1   Distant metastasis microscopically confirmed

Note

pM0 and pMX are not valid categories.

Summary

Prostate	
T1	Not palpable
T1a	≤ 5%
T1b	> 5%
T1c	Needle biopsy
T2	Palpable and confined within prostate
T2a	≤ half of one lobe
T2b	> half of one lobe
T2c	Both lobes
T3	Through prostatic capsule
T3a	Extraprostatic extension including microscopic bladder neck involvement
T3b	Seminal vesicle(s)
T4	Fixed or invades adjacent structures other than seminal vesicles: sphincter externus, rectum, levator muscles, pelvic wall
N1	Regional lymph node(s)
M1a	Non-regional lymph node(s)
M1b	Bone(s)
M1c	Other site(s)

TESTIS (ICD-O-3 C62) (FIG. 489)

Rules for Classification

The classification applies only to germ cell tumours of the testis. There should be histological confirmation of the disease and division of cases by histological type. Histopathological grading is not applicable.

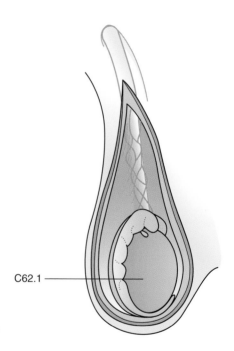

C62.1

Fig. 489

353

Regional Lymph Nodes (Fig. 490)

The regional lymph nodes are the abdominal para-aortic (periaortic), preaortic, interaortocaval, precaval, paracaval, retrocaval, and retroaortic nodes. Nodes along the spermatic vein should be considered regional. Laterality does not affect the N classification. The intrapelvic nodes and the inguinal nodes are considered regional after scrotal or inguinal surgery.

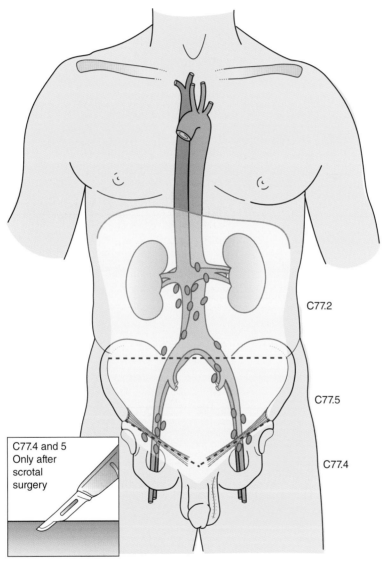

C77.2

C77.5

C77.4 and 5
Only after
scrotal
surgery

C77.4

Fig. 490

TNM Clinical Classification

T – Primary Tumour

Except for pTis and pT4, where radical orchiectomy is not always necessary for classification purposes, the extent of the primary tumour is classified after radical orchiectomy; see pT. In other circumstances, TX is used if no radical orchiectomy has been performed.

N – Regional Lymph Nodes

NX   Regional lymph nodes cannot be assessed
N0   No regional lymph node metastasis
N1   Metastasis with a lymph node mass 2 cm or less in greatest dimension or multiple lymph nodes, none more than 2 cm in greatest dimension (Figs. 491, 492, 493, 494, 495)

N1

pN1

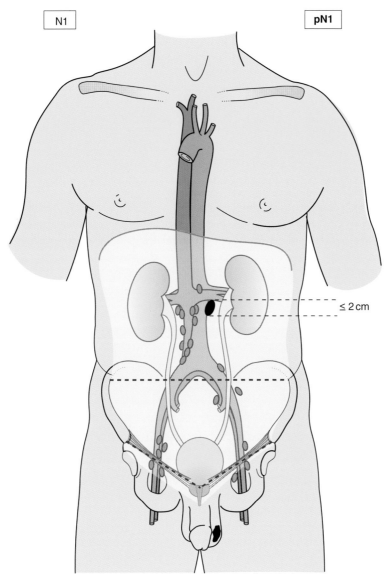

≤ 2 cm

Fig. 491

N1   pN1

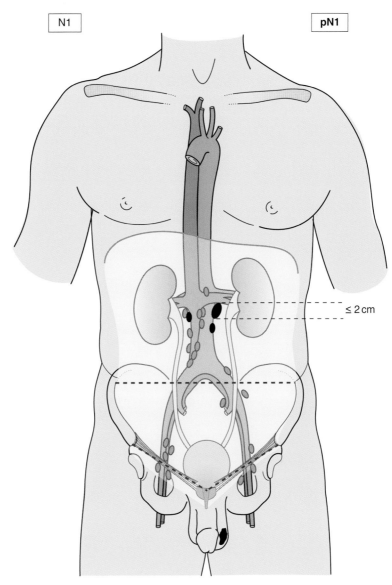

≤ 2 cm

Fig. 492

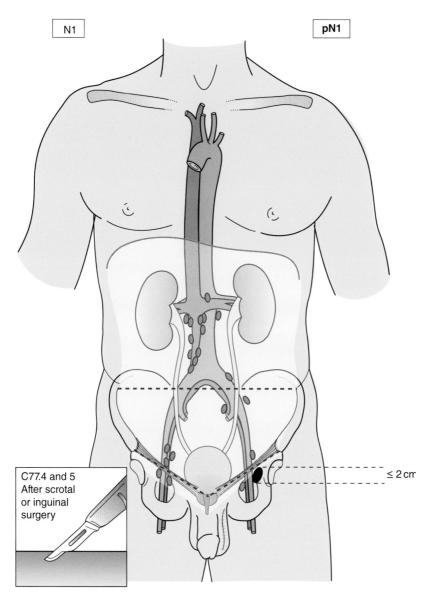

N1

pN1

C77.4 and 5
After scrotal
or inguinal
surgery

≤ 2 cm

Fig. 493

N1

pN1

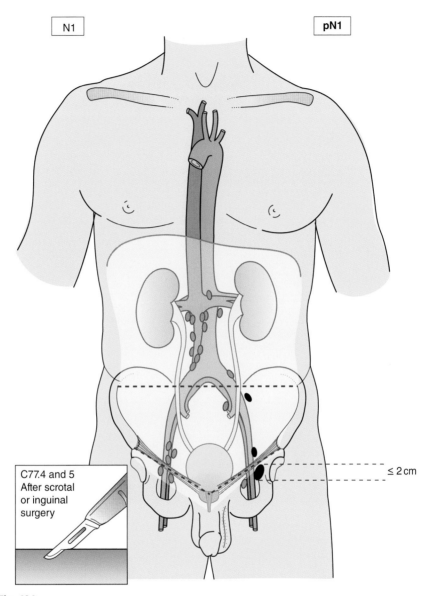

C77.4 and 5
After scrotal
or inguinal
surgery

≤ 2 cm

Fig. 494

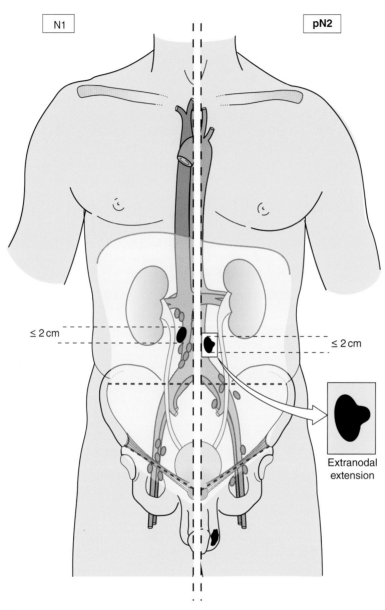

N1

pN2

≤ 2 cm

≤ 2 cm

Extranodal
extension

Fig. 495

N2   Metastasis with a lymph node mass more than 2 cm but not more than 5 cm in greatest dimension, or multiple lymph nodes, any one mass more than 2 cm but not more than 5 cm in greatest dimension (Figs. 496, 497)

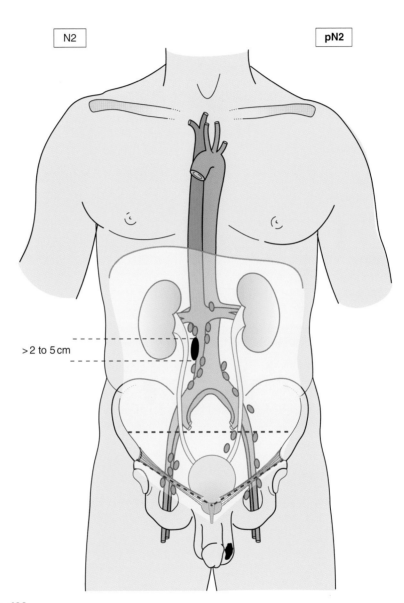

Fig. 496

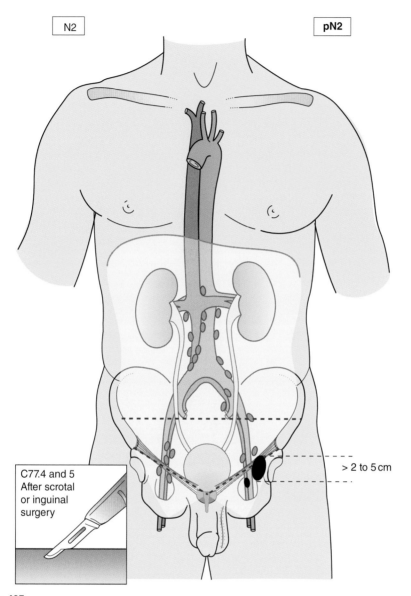

N2

pN2

C77.4 and 5
After scrotal
or inguinal
surgery

> 2 to 5 cm

Fig. 497

N3   Metastasis with a lymph node mass more than 5 cm in greatest dimension (Figs. 498, 499, 500, 501)

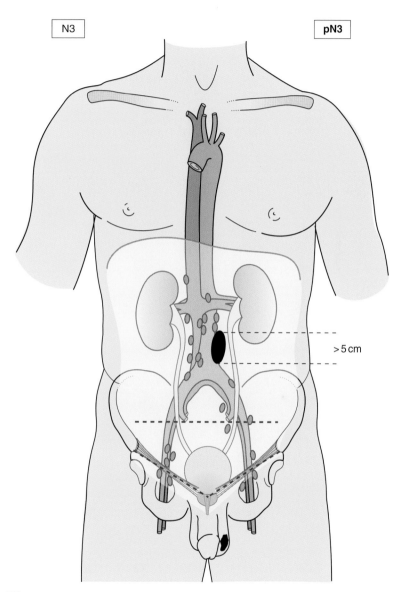

Fig. 498

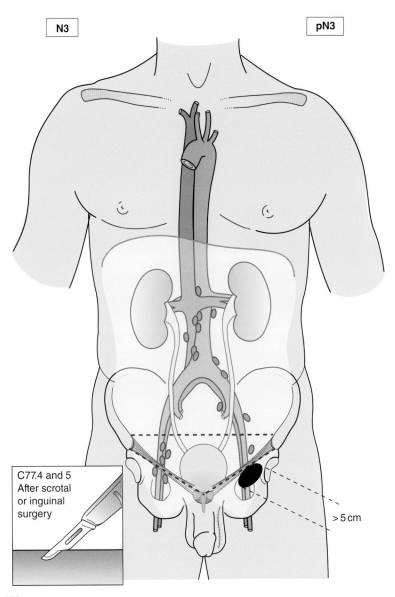

N3

pN3

C77.4 and 5
After scrotal
or inguinal
surgery

> 5 cm

Fig. 499

N3

pN3

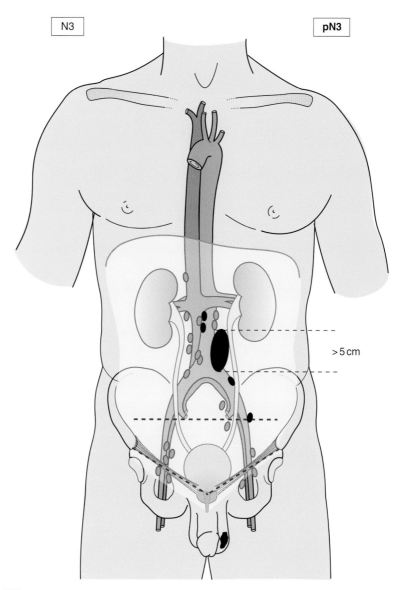

>5 cm

Fig. 500

N3

pN3

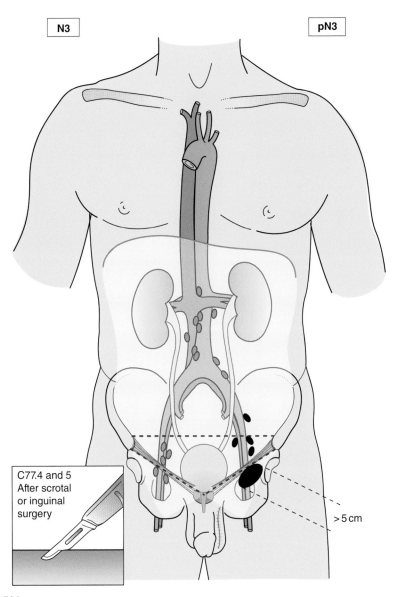

C77.4 and 5
After scrotal
or inguinal
surgery

> 5 cm

Fig. 501

M – Distant Metastasis

M0   No distant metastasis
M1   Distant metastasis
      M1a   Non-regional lymph node(s) or lung metastasis
      M1b   Distant metastasis other than non-regional lymph nodes and lung

pTNM Pathological Classification

pT – Primary Tumour

pTX   Primary tumour cannot be assessed (see T – Primary Tumour, above)
pT0   No evidence of primary tumour (e.g., histologic scar in testis)
pTis   Intratubular germ cell neoplasia (carcinoma in situ)

pT1   Tumour limited to testis and epididymis without vascular/lymphatic invasion; tumour may invade tunica albuginea but not tunica vaginalis (Fig. 502)
pT2   Tumour limited to testis and epididymis with vascular/lymphatic invasion (Fig. 502), or tumour extending through tunica albuginea with involvement of tunica vaginalis (Fig. 503)
pT3   Tumour invades spermatic cord with or without vascular/lymphatic invasion (Fig. 504)
pT4   Tumour invades scrotum with or without vascular/ lymphatic invasion (Fig. 505)

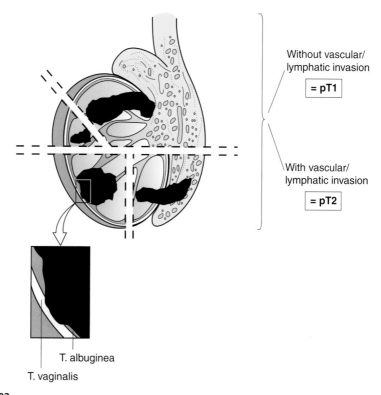

Fig. 502

pT2

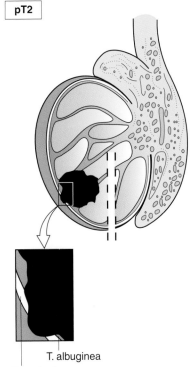

T. albuginea

Fig. 503   T. vaginalis

pT3

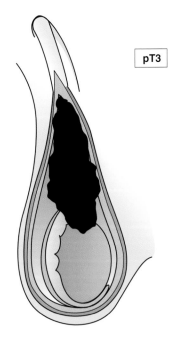

Fig. 504

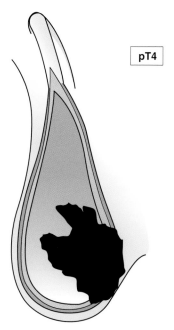

pT4

Fig. 505

pN – Regional Lymph Nodes

pNX   Regional lymph nodes cannot be assessed

pN0   No regional lymph node metastasis

pN1   Metastasis with a lymph node mass 2 cm or less in greatest dimension and 5 or fewer positive nodes, none more than 2 cm in greatest dimension (Figs. 491, 492, 493, 494)

pN2   Metastasis with a lymph node mass (Figs. 495, 496, 497) more than 2 cm but not more than 5 cm in greatest dimension; or more than 5 nodes positive, none more than 5 cm; or evidence of extranodal extension of tumour (Fig. 495)

pN3   Metastasis with a lymph node mass more than 5 cm in greatest dimension (Figs. 498, 499, 500, 501)

pM – Distant Metastasis

pM1   Distant metastasis microscopically confirmed

Note

pM0 and pMX are not valid categories.

Summary

Testis			
pTis	Intratubular		
pT1	Testis and epididymis, no vascular/lymphatic invasion		
pT2	Testis and epididymis with vascular/lymphatic invasion or tunica vaginalis		
pT3	Spermatic cord		
pT4	Scrotum		
N1	≤ 2 cm	pN1	≤ 2 cm and ≤ 5 nodes
N2	> 2 to 5 cm	pN2	> 2 to 5 cm or > 5 nodes or extranodal extension
N3	> 5 cm	pN3	> 5 cm
M1a	Non-regional lymph nodes or lung		
M1b	Other sites		

KIDNEY (ICD-O-3 C64) (FIG. 506)

Rules for Classification

The classification applies only to renal cell carcinoma. There should be histological confirmation of the disease.

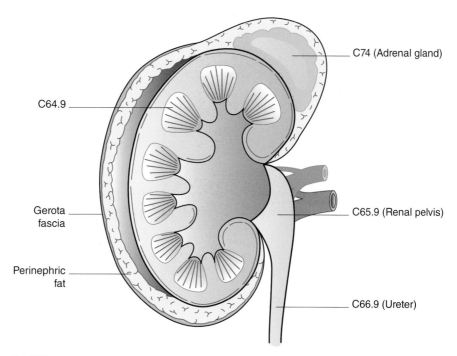

Fig. 506

Regional Lymph Nodes (Fig. 507)

The regional lymph nodes are the hilar, abdominal para-aortic, and paracaval nodes. Laterality does not affect the N categories.

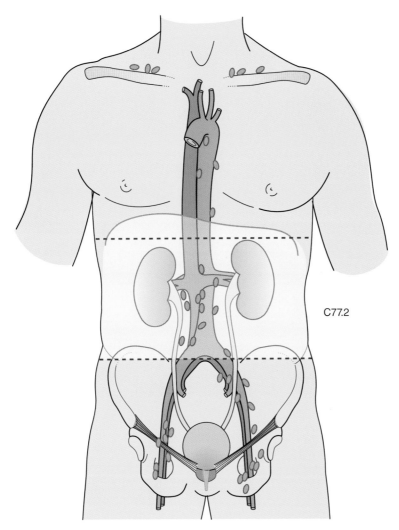

C77.2

Fig. 507

TNM Clinical Classification

T – Primary Tumour

TX   Primary tumour cannot be assessed

T0   No evidence of primary tumour

T1   Tumour 7 cm or less in greatest dimension, limited to the kidney

       T1a   Tumour 4 cm or less (Fig. 508)

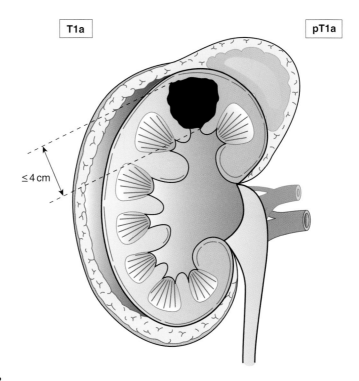

T1a   pT1a

≤ 4 cm

Fig. 508

T1b Tumour more than 4 cm but not more than 7 cm (Fig. 509)

T2 Tumour more than 7 cm in greatest dimension, limited to the kidney (Fig. 510)

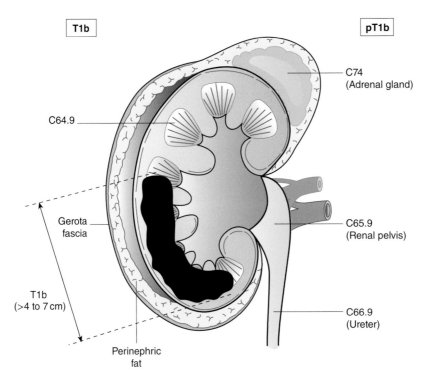

Fig. 509

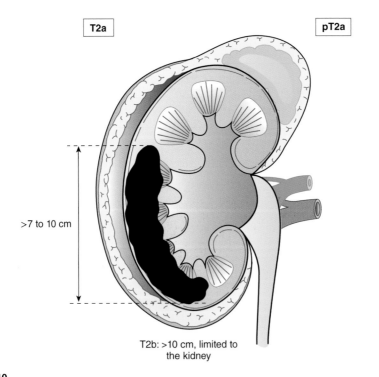

Fig. 510

T2a   Tumour more than 7 cm but not more than 10 cm

T2b   Tumour more than 10 cm, limited to the kidney

T3   Tumour extends into major veins or perinephric tissues but not into the ipsilateral adrenal gland and not beyond Gerota fascia

T3a   Tumour extends into the renal vein or its segmental branches, or tumour invades the pelvicalyceal system, or tumour invades perirenal and/or renal sinus fat (peripelvic fat) but not beyond Gerota fascia (Fig. 511)

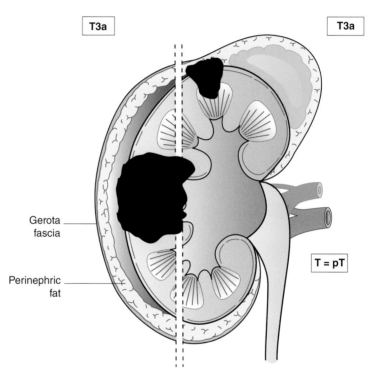

Fig. 511

T3b   Tumour extends into vena cava below diaphragm (Fig. 512)

T3c   Tumour extends into vena cava above the diaphragm or invades the wall
of the vena cava (Fig. 513)

T4   Tumour invades beyond Gerota fascia (including contiguous extension into the
ipsilateral adrenal gland) (Figs. 514a, 514b)

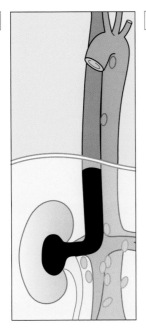

Fig. 512

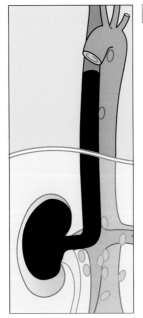

Fig. 513

(a)

T4

pT4

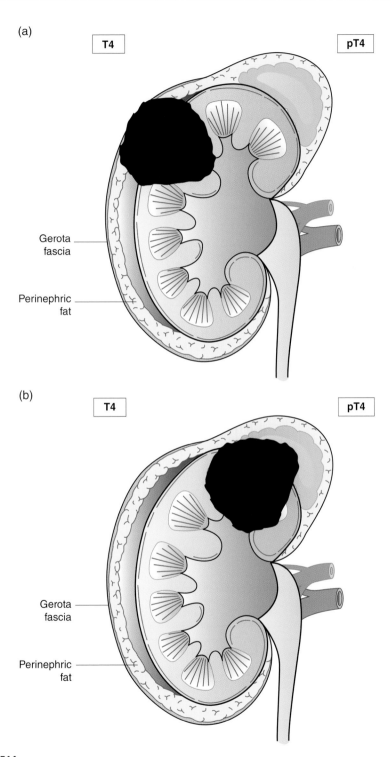

Gerota
fascia

Perinephric
fat

(b)

T4

pT4

Gerota
fascia

Perinephric
fat

Fig. 514

N – Regional Lymph Nodes

NX   Regional lymph nodes cannot be assessed
N0   No regional lymph node metastasis
N1   Metastasis in regional lymph node(s) (Fig. 515)

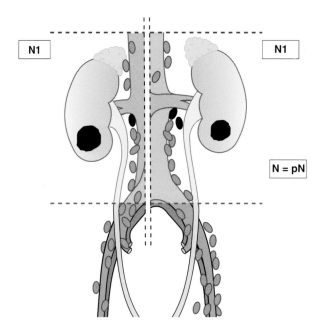

Fig. 515

M – Distant Metastasis

M0   No distant metastasis
M1   Distant metastasis

pTNM Pathological Classification

The pT and pN categories correspond to the T and N categories.

pM1   Distant metastasis microscopically confirmed

Note
pM0 and pMX are not valid categories.

Summary

Kidney	
T1	≤ 7 cm; limited to the kidney
T1a	≤ 4 cm
T1b	> 4 cm
T2	> 7 cm; limited to the kidney
T2a	> 7 to 10 cm
T2b	> 10 cm
T3	Major veins, perinephric tissues but not into the ipsilateral adrenal gland and not beyond Gerota fascia
T3a	Renal vein or its segmental branches or pelvicalyceal system, perinephric and/or renal sinus fat
T3b	Vena cava below diaphragm
T3c	Vena cava above diaphragm
T4	Beyond Gerota fascia, ipsilateral adrenal gland
N1	Regional
M1	Distant

RENAL PELVIS AND URETER

(ICD-O-3 C65, C66)

Rules for Classification

The classification applies to carcinomas. Papilloma is excluded. There should be histological or cytological confirmation of the disease.

Anatomical Sites (Fig. 506)

1. Renal pelvis (C65)
2. Ureter (C66)

Regional Lymph Nodes (Fig. 507)

The regional lymph nodes are the hilar, abdominal para-aortic, and paracaval nodes and, for ureter, intrapelvic nodes. Laterality does not affect the N classification.

TNM Clinical Classification

T – Primary Tumour

TX   Primary tumour cannot be assessed
T0   No evidence of primary tumour
Ta   Noninvasive papillary carcinoma (Fig. 516)
Tis   Carcinoma in situ

T1   Tumour invades subepithelial connective tissue (Fig. 516)
T2   Tumour invades muscularis (Fig. 516)
T3   *(Renal pelvis)* Tumour invades beyond muscularis into peripelvic fat or renal parenchyma (Fig. 517)
        (Ureter) Tumour invades beyond muscularis into periureteric fat (Fig. 517)

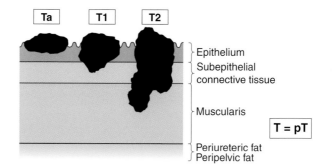

Fig. 516

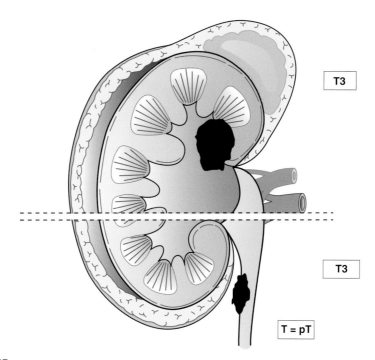

Fig. 517

T4   Tumour invades adjacent organs (Figs. 518, 519) or through the kidney into perinephric fat (Fig. 520)

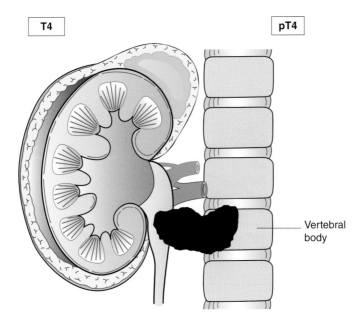

Fig. 518

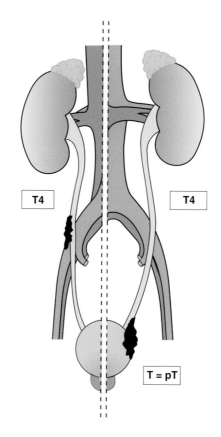

T4

T4

T = pT

Fig. 519

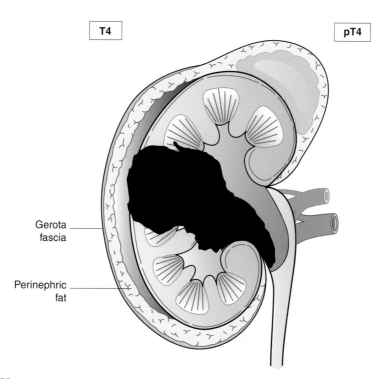

T4

pT4

Gerota
fascia

Perinephric
fat

Fig. 520

N – Regional Lymph Nodes

NX   Regional lymph nodes cannot be assessed

N0   No regional lymph node metastasis

N1   Metastasis in a single lymph node 2 cm or less in greatest dimension (Fig. 521)

N2   Metastasis in a single lymph node more than 2 cm or multiple lymph nodes (Figs. 522, 523)

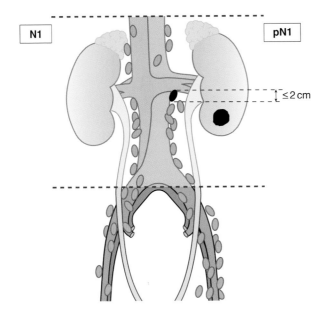

Fig. 521

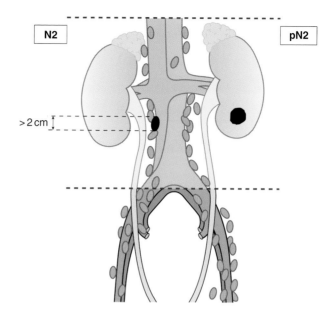

Fig. 522

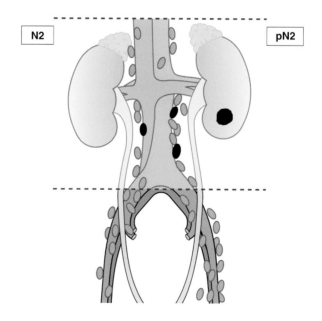

Fig. 523

M – Distant Metastasis

M0   No distant metastasis
M1   Distant metastasis

pTNM Pathological Classification

The pT and pN categories correspond to the T and N categories.

pM1   Distant metastasis microscopically confirmed

Note
pM0 and pMX are not valid categories.

Summary

Renal Pelvis and Ureter	
Ta	Noninvasive, papillary
Tis	In situ
T1	Subepithelial connective tissue
T2	Muscularis
T3	Beyond muscularis
T4	Adjacent organs, perinephric fat
N1	Single ≤ 2 cm
N2	Single > 2 cm or multiple
M1	Distant

URINARY BLADDER (ICD-O-3 C67)

Rules for Classification

The classification applies to carcinomas. Papilloma is excluded. There should be histological or cytological confirmation of the disease.

Anatomical Subsites (Fig. 524)

1. Trigone (C67.0)
2. Dome (C67.1)
3. Lateral wall (C67.2)
4. Anterior wall (C67.3)
5. Posterior wall (C67.4)
6. Bladder neck (C67.5)
7. Ureteric orifice (C67.6)
8. Urachus (C67.7)

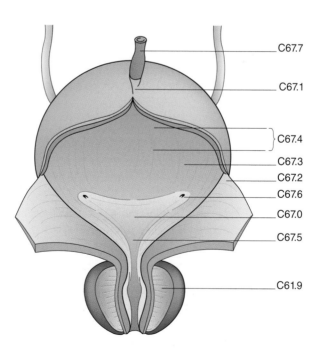

Fig. 524

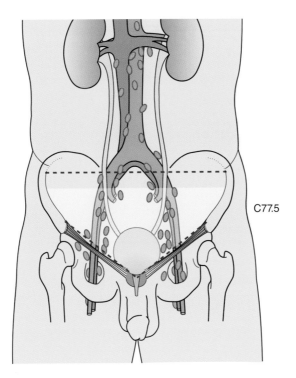

C77.5

Fig. 525

Regional Lymph Nodes (Fig. 525)

The regional lymph nodes are the nodes of the true pelvis, which essentially are the pelvic nodes below the bifurcation and those along the common iliac arteries. Laterality does not affect the N classification.

TNM Clinical Classification

T – Primary Tumour (Fig. 526)

The suffix (m) should be added to the appropriate T category to indicate multiple tumours. The suffix (is) may be added to any T to indicate presence of associated carcinoma in situ.

TX	Primary tumour cannot be assessed
T0	No evidence of primary tumour
Ta	Noninvasive papillary carcinoma
Tis	Carcinoma in situ: "flat tumour"
T1	Tumour invades subepithelial connective tissue
T2	Tumour invades muscularis propria
	T2a Tumour invades muscularis propria (inner half)
	T2b Tumour invades deep muscularis propria (outer half)

T3   Tumour invades perivesical tissue:

      T3a   microscopically

      T3b   macroscopically (extravesical mass)

T4   Tumour invades any of the following: prostate stroma, seminal vesicles, uterus, vagina, pelvic wall, abdominal wall

      T4a   Tumour invades prostate stroma, seminal vesicles, uterus, or vagina

      T4b   Tumour invades pelvic wall or abdominal wall

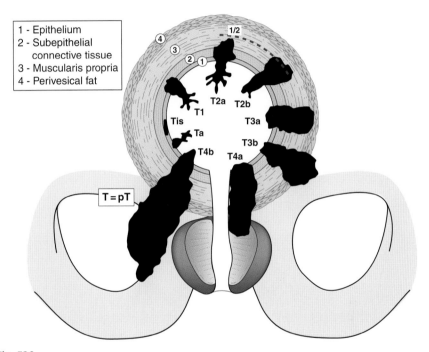

1 - Epithelium
2 - Subepithelial
    connective tissue
3 - Muscularis propria
4 - Perivesical fat

T = pT

Fig. 526

N – Regional Lymph Nodes

NX   Regional lymph nodes cannot be assessed

N0   No regional lymph node metastasis

N1   Metastasis in a single lymph node in the true pelvis (hypogastric, obturator, external iliac, or presacral) (Fig. 527)

N2   Metastasis in multiple regional lymph nodes in the true pelvis (hypogastric, obturator, external iliac, or presacral) (Fig. 528)

N3   Metastasis in a common iliac lymph node(s) (Fig. 529)

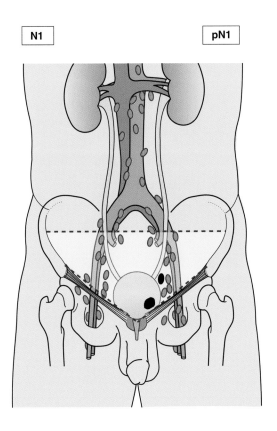

Fig. 527

N2

pN2

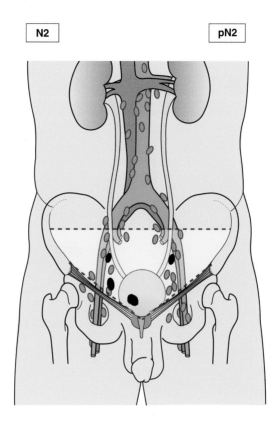

Fig. 528

N3   pN3

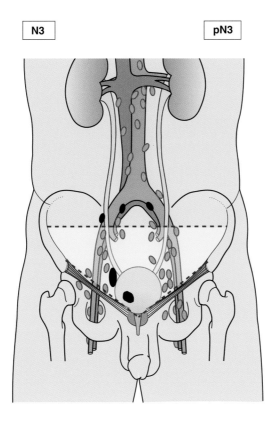

Fig. 529

M – Distant Metastasis

M0   No distant metastasis
M1a   Non-regional lymph nodes
M1b   Other distant metastasis

pTNM Pathological Classification

The pT and pN categories correspond to the T and N categories.

pM1a   Non-regional lymph nodes
pM1b   Other distant metastasis

Note
pM0 and pMX are not valid categories.

Summary

Urinary Bladder	
Ta	Noninvasive papillary
Tis	In situ: "flat tumour"
T1	Subepithelial connective tissue
T2	Muscularis propria
T2a	Inner half
T2b	Outer half
T3	Perivesical tissue
T3a	Microscopically
T3b	Extravesical mass
T4	Prostate, uterus, vagina, pelvic wall, abdominal wall
T4a	Prostate, uterus, vagina
T4b	Pelvic wall, abdominal wall
N1	Single
N2	Multiple
N3	Common iliac
M1	Distant

URETHRA

Rules for Classification

The classification applies to carcinomas of the urethra (ICD-O-3 C68.0) and transitional cell carcinomas of the prostate (ICD-O-3 C61.9) and prostatic urethra. There should be histological or cytological confirmation of the disease.

Regional Lymph Nodes (Fig. 490)

The regional lymph nodes are the inguinal and the pelvic nodes. Laterality does not affect the N classification.

TNM Clinical Classification

T – Primary Tumour

TX   Primary tumour cannot be assessed
T0   No evidence of primary tumour

Urethra (Male and Female)

Ta   Noninvasive papillary, polypoid, or verrucous carcinoma (Figs. 530, 531)
Tis   Carcinoma in situ

T1   Tumour invades subepithelial connective tissue (Figs. 530, 532)
T2   Tumour invades any of the following: corpus spongiosum, prostate, periurethral muscle (Figs. 530, 533, 534)

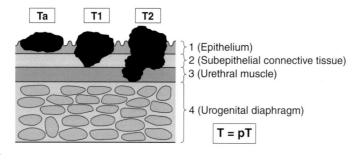

Fig. 530

Ta   pTa

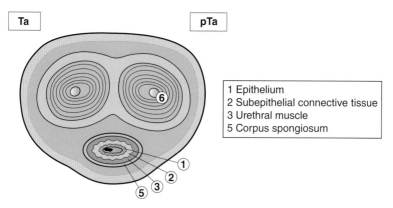

1 Epithelium
2 Subepithelial connective tissue
3 Urethral muscle
5 Corpus spongiosum

Fig. 531

T1   pT1

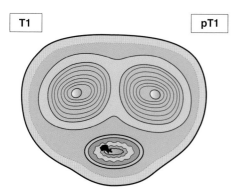

Fig. 532

T2   pT2

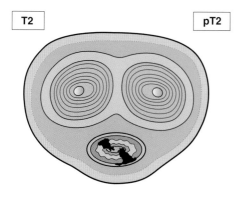

Fig. 533

T2   T2

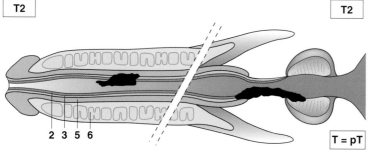

2 Subepithelial connective
  tissue
3 Urethral muscle
5 Corpus spongiosum
6 Corpus cavernosum

T = pT

Fig. 534

T3   Tumour invades any of the following: corpus cavernosum, beyond prostatic capsule, bladder neck (extraprostatic extension) (Figs. 535, 536, 537)

T4   Tumour invades other adjacent organs (invasion of the bladder) (Fig. 538)

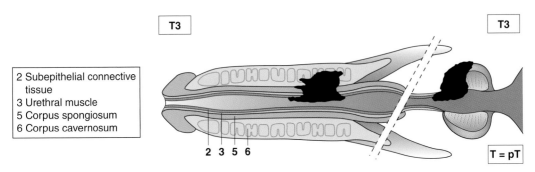

T3

2 Subepithelial connective tissue
3 Urethral muscle
5 Corpus spongiosum
6 Corpus cavernosum

2 3 5 6

T3

T = pT

Fig. 535

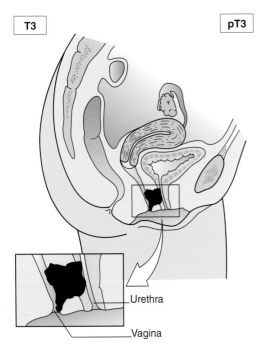

T3

pT3

Urethra

Vagina

Fig. 536

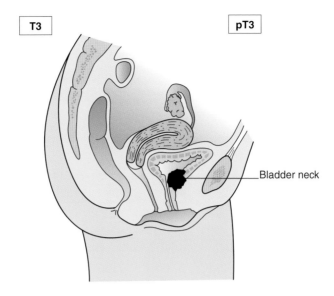

Fig. 537

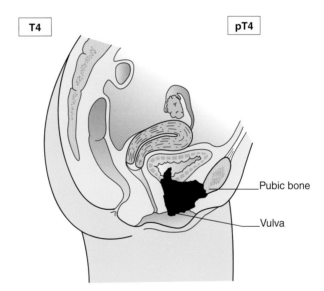

Fig. 538

Prostatic urethra

Tis   Carcinoma in situ, involving prostatic urethra, periurethral or prostatic ducts without stromal invasion (Figs. 539, 540)

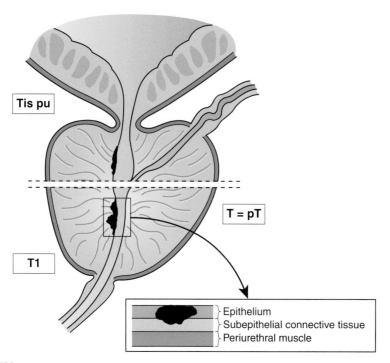

Fig. 539

T1   Tumour invades subepithelial connective tissue (for tumours involving prostatic urethra only) (Figs. 540, 541)

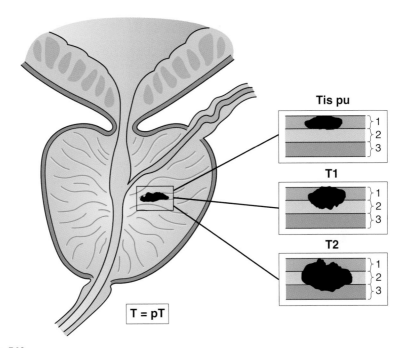

Fig. 540

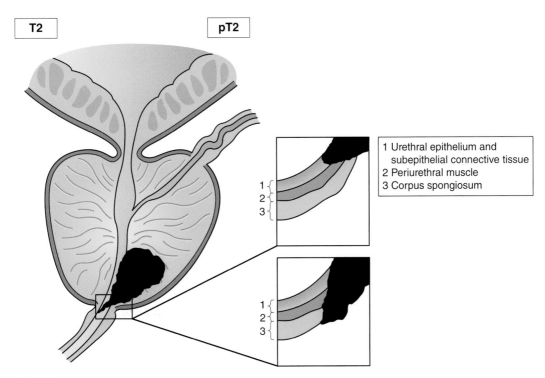

Fig. 541

T2   Tumour invades any of the following: prostatic stroma, corpus spongiosum, periurethral muscle (Figs. 540, 541)

T3   Tumour invades any of the following: corpus cavernosum, beyond prostatic capsule, bladder neck (extraprostatic extension) (Fig. 542)

T4   Tumour invades other adjacent organs (invasion of bladder) (Fig. 543)

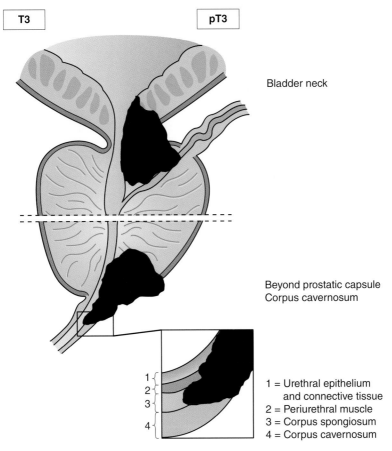

Fig. 542

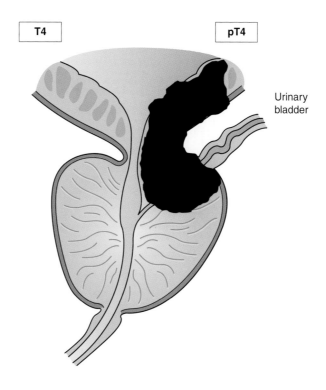

T4   pT4

Urinary
bladder

Fig. 543

N – Regional Lymph Nodes

NX   Regional lymph nodes cannot be assessed
N0   No regional lymph node metastasis
N1   Metastasis in a single lymph node (Fig. 544)
N2   Metastasis in multiple lymph nodes (Fig. 545)

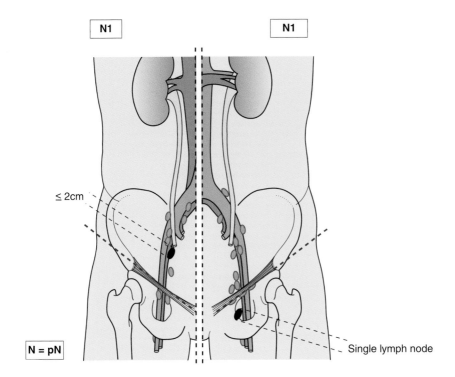

N1

N1

≤ 2cm

N = pN

Single lymph node

Fig. 544

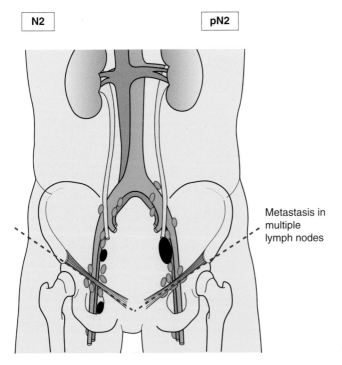

N2

pN2

Metastasis in
multiple
lymph nodes

Fig. 545

M – Distant Metastasis

M0   No distant metastasis
M1   Distant metastasis

pTNM Pathological Classification

The pT, pN, and pM categories correspond to the T, N, and M categories.

pM1   Distant metastasis microscopically confirmed

Note
pM0 and pMX are not valid categories.

Summary

	Urethra
Ta	Noninvasive papillary, polypoid, verrucous
Tis	In situ
T1	Subepithelial connective tissue
T2	Corpus spongiosum, prostate, periurethral muscle
T3	Corpus cavernosum, beyond prostatic capsule (extraprostatic extension), bladder neck
T4	Other adjacent organs (bladder)
	Prostatic Urethra
Tis	Carcinoma in situ, involving prostatic urethra, periurethral or prostatic ducts without stromal invasion
T1	Subepithelial connective tissue
T2	Prostatic stroma, corpus spongiosum, periurethral muscle
T3	Corpus cavernosum, beyond prostatic capsule, bladder neck (extraprostatic extension)
T4	Other adjacent organs (bladder)
N1	Single
N2	Multiple
M1	Distant

ADRENAL CORTEX TUMOURS (ICD-O-3 C74.0)

Rules for Classification

This classification applies only to carcinomas of the adrenal cortex. It does not apply to tumours of the adrenal medulla or sarcomas.

Regional Lymph Nodes

The regional lymph nodes are the hilar, abdominal para-aortic, and paracaval nodes. Laterality does not affect the N categories.

TNM Clinical Classification

T – Primary Tumour

TX   Primary tumour cannot be assessed

T0   No evidence of primary tumour

T1   Tumour 5 cm or less in greatest dimension, no extra-adrenal invasion (Fig. 546)

T2   Tumour greater than 5 cm, no extra-adrenal invasion (Fig. 547)

T3   Tumour of any size with local invasion, but not invading adjacent organs* (Fig. 548)

T4   Tumour of any size with invasion of adjacent organs* (Fig. 549)

Note

*Adjacent organs include kidney, diaphragm, great vessels (renal vein or vena cava), pancreas, and liver.

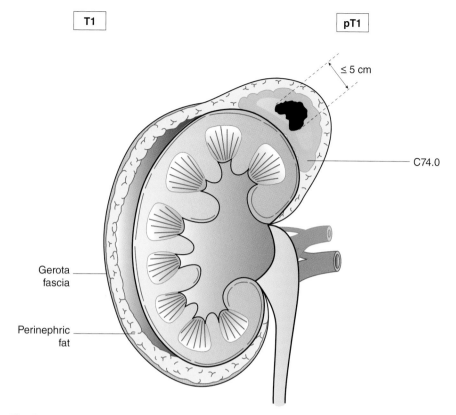

Fig. 546

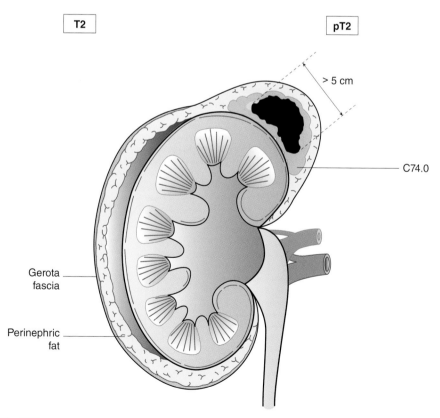

Fig. 547

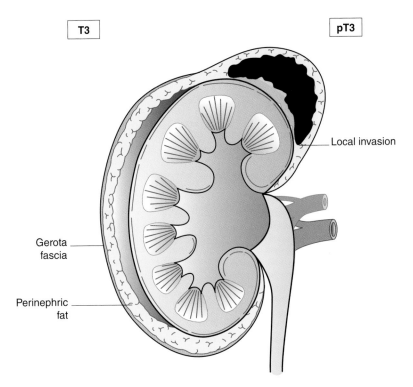

T3   pT3

Local invasion

Gerota fascia

Perinephric fat

Fig. 548

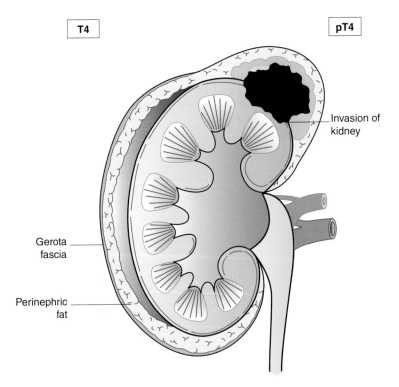

T4   pT4

Invasion of kidney

Gerota fascia

Perinephric fat

Fig. 549

N – Regional Lymph Nodes

NX   Regional lymph nodes cannot be assessed
N0   No regional lymph node metastasis
N1   Metastasis in regional lymph node(s)

M – Distant Metastasis

M0   No distant metastasis
M1   Distant metastasis

pTNM Pathological Classification

The pT, pN, and pM categories correspond to the T, N, and M categories.

pM1   Distant metastasis microscopically confirmed

Note
pM0 and pMX are not valid categories.

Summary

Adrenal Cortical Carcinoma	
T1	≤ 5 cm, no extra-adrenal invasion
T2	> 5 cm, no extra-adrenal invasion
T3	Local invasion
T4	Adjacent organs
N1	Regional
M1	Distant

HODGKIN LYMPHOMA

Introductory Notes

The current staging classification for Hodgkin Lymphoma is a modification of the Ann Arbor classification first adopted in 1971. Over the past 50 years the practice has changed, making the previously used staging laparotomy and the resulting pathological staging classification obsolete. The consensus conference that took place in 2012 in Lugano suggested an even more simplified system, putting together Stages I and II as Limited Stage and Stages III and IV as Advanced Stage lymphoma. The Lugano Classification, a modification of the Ann Arbor classification, has been published and accepted by the UICC.[1]

Clinical Staging (cS)

This is determined by history, clinical examination, imaging, blood analysis and the initial biopsy report. Bone marrow biopsy must be taken from a clinically or radiologically non-involved area of bone.

Liver Involvement

Clinical evidence of liver involvement must include either enlargement of the liver and at least an abnormal serum alkaline phosphatase level and two different liver function test abnormalities, or an abnormal liver demonstrated by imaging and one abnormal liver function test.

---

[1]Cheson BD, Fisher RI, Barrington SF, et al. (2014) Recommendations for initial evaluation, staging, and response assessment of Hodgkin and non-Hodgkin lymphoma: the Lugano classification. *J Clin Oncol* 32:3059–3068.

Spleen Involvement

Clinical evidence of spleen involvement is accepted if there is palpable enlargement of the spleen confirmed by imaging.

Lymphatic and Extralymphatic Disease

The lymphatic structures are as follows:
- Lymph nodes
- Waldeyer ring
- Spleen
- Appendix
- Thymus
- Peyer patches

The lymph nodes are grouped into regions and one or more (2, 3, etc.) may be involved. The spleen is designated S and extralymphatic organs or sites E.

Lung Involvement

Lung involvement limited to one lobe, or perihilar extension associated with ipsilateral lymphadenopathy, or unilateral pleural effusion with or without lung involvement but with hilar lymphadenopathy is considered as *localized* extralymphatic disease.

Liver Involvement

Liver involvement is always considered as *diffuse* extralymphatic disease.

Clinical Stages (cS)

Limited Stage

Stage I

Involvement of a single lymph node region (I) (Figs. 550, 551, 552, 553) or localized involvement of a single extralymphatic organ or site (IE) (Fig. 554).

S: I

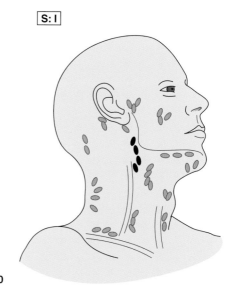

Fig. 550

S: I

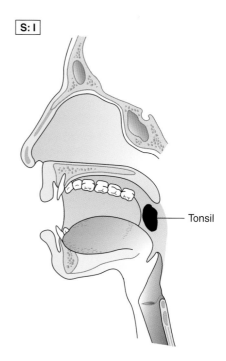

Tonsil

Fig. 551

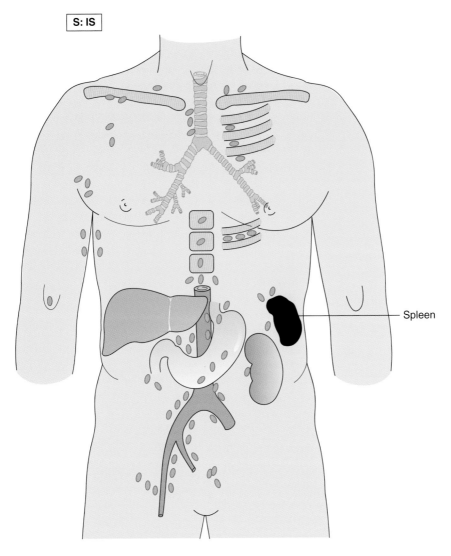

S: IS

Spleen

Fig. 552

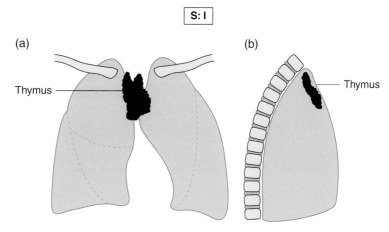

Fig. 553

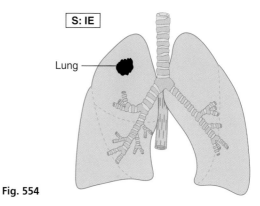

Fig. 554

Stage II

Involvement of two or more lymph node regions on the same side of the diaphragm (II) (Fig. 555), or localized involvement of a single extralymphatic organ or site and its regional lymph node(s) with or without involvement of other lymph node regions on the same side of the diaphragm (IIE) (Fig. 556).

S: II

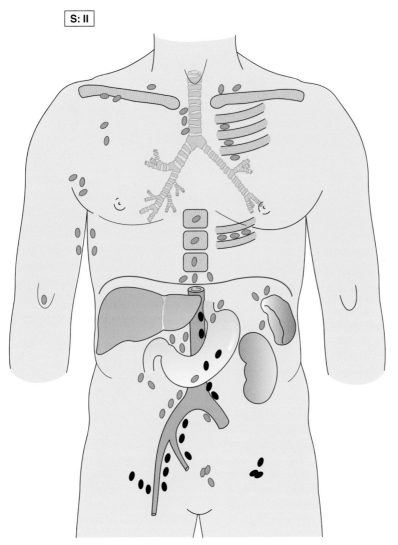

Fig. 555

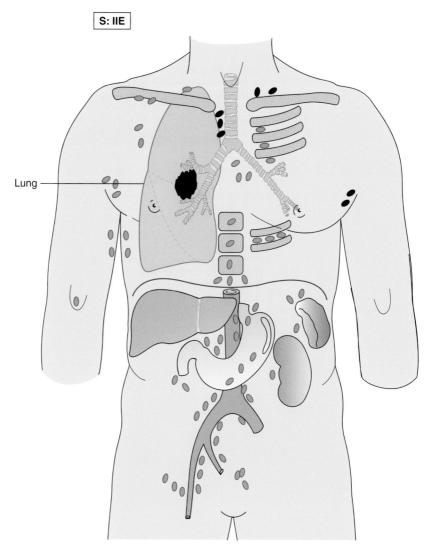

S: IIE

Lung

Fig. 556

Bulky Stage II

Stage II disease with a single nodal mass greater than 10 cm in maximum dimension or greater than a third of the thoracic diameter as assessed on CT (Figs. 557, 558, 559).

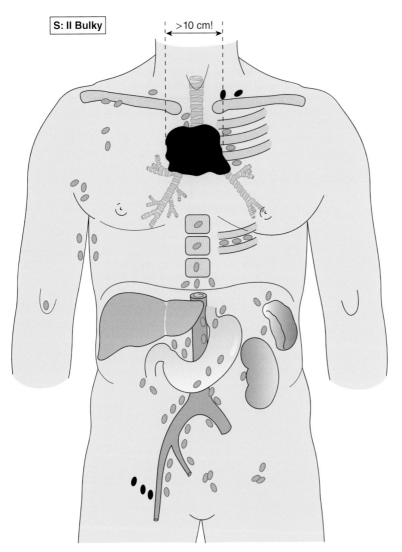

Fig. 557

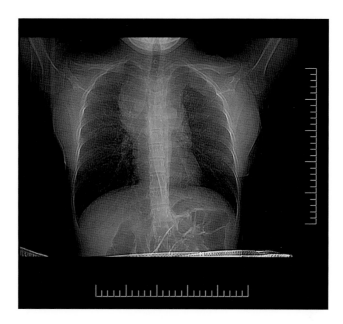

Fig. 558

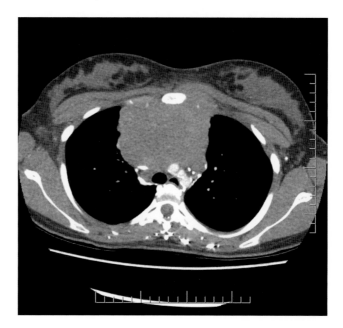

Fig. 559

Advanced Stage

Stage III

Involvement of lymph node regions on both sides of the diaphragm (III) (Fig. 560), which may also be accompanied by localized involvement of an associated extralymphatic organ or site (IIIE) (Fig. 561), or by involvement of the spleen (IIIS), or both (IIIE + S) (Fig. 562).

S: III

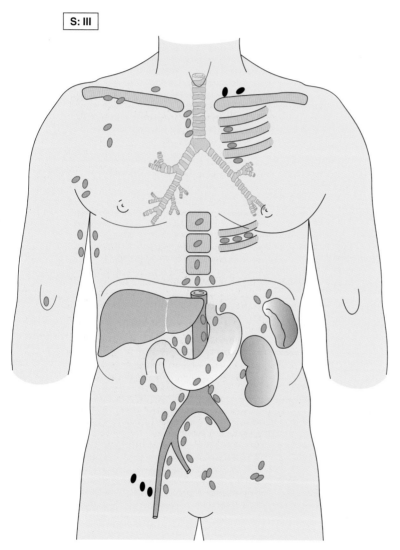

Fig. 560

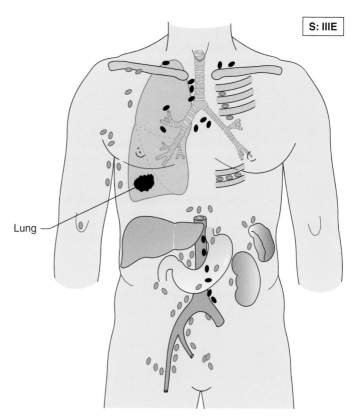

Fig. 561

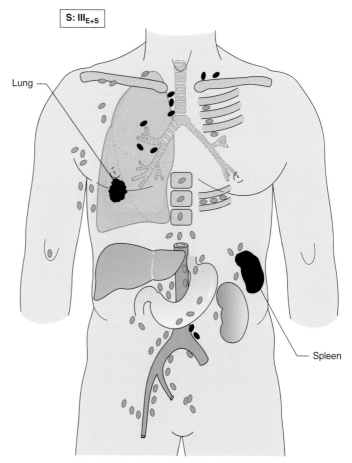

Fig. 562

Stage IV

Disseminated (multifocal) involvement of one or more extralymphatic organs, with or without associated lymph node involvement (Figs. 563, 564); or non-contiguous extralymphatic organ involvement with involvement of lymph node regions on the same or both sides of the diaphragm (Fig. 565).

Note
The site of Stage IV disease is identified further by specifying sites according to the notations listed above.

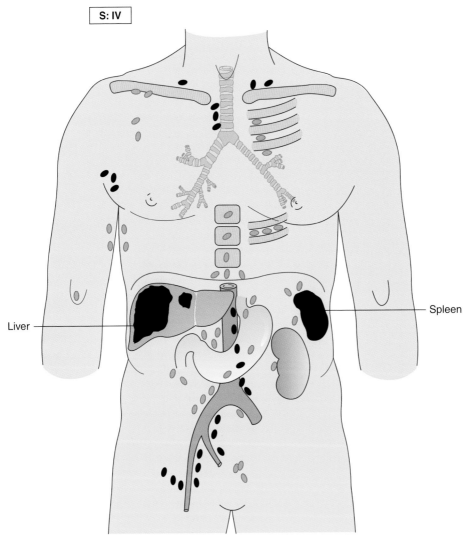

Fig. 563

S: IV

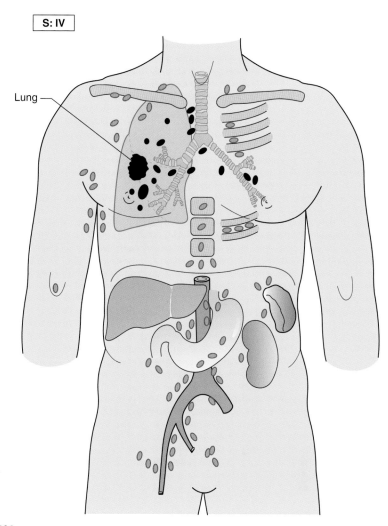

Lung

Fig. 564

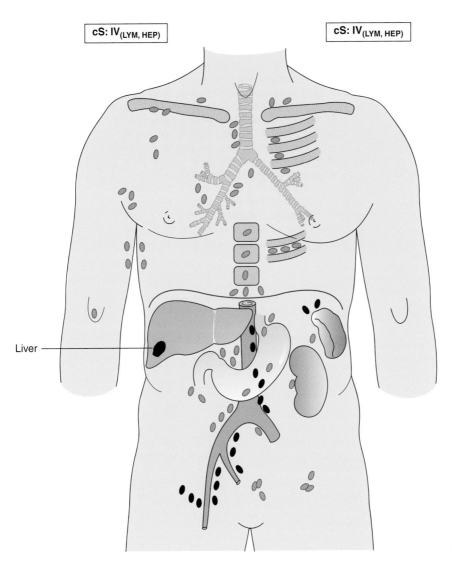

cS: IV$_{(LYM, HEP)}$

cS: IV$_{(LYM, HEP)}$

Liver

Fig. 565

A and B Classification (Symptoms)

Each stage should be divided into A and B according to the absence or presence of defined general symptoms. These are:
1. Unexplained weight loss of more than 10% of the usual body weight in the 6 months prior to first attendance
2. Unexplained fever with temperature above 38 °C
3. Night sweats

Note

Pruritus alone does not qualify for B classification, nor does a short, febrile illness associated with a known infection.

Summary

Stage		Hodgkin Lymphoma	Substage
Stage I	Limited	Single node region	I
		Localized single extralymphatic organ/site	IE
Stage II	Limited	Two or more node regions same side of diaphragm	II
		Localized single extralymphatic organ/site with its regional nodes	IIE
		± other node regions same side of diaphragm	
Stage III	Advanced	Node regions both sides of diaphragm	III
		+ localized single extralymphatic organ/site	IIIE
		Spleen	IIIS
		Both	IIIE + S
Stage IV	Advanced	Diffuse or multifocal involvement of extralymphatic organ(s) ± regional nodes; isolated extralymphatic organ and non-regional nodes	
All stages		Without weight loss/fever/sweats	A
divided		With weight loss/fever/sweats	B

NON-HODGKIN LYMPHOMAS

The staging classification for non-Hodgkin lymphomas is the same as for Hodgkin lymphomas.

INDEX

TNM Atlas: Illustrated Guide to the TNM Classification of Malignant Tumours, Seventh Edition.
Edited by James D. Brierley, Hisao Asamura, Elisabeth Van Eycken, and Brian Rous.
© 2021 by UICC. Published 2021 by John Wiley & Sons Ltd.